A PHILOSOPHER GOES TO THE DOCTOR

This book sheds light on important philosophical assumptions made by professionals working in clinical and research medicine. In doing so, it aims to make explicit how active philosophy is in medicine and shows how this awareness can result in better and more informed medical research and practice.

It examines: what features make something a scientific discipline; the inherent tensions between understanding medicine as a research science and as a healing practice; how the "replication crisis" in medical research asks us to rethink the structure of knowledge production in our modern world; whether explanations have any real scientific values; the uncertainties about probabilistic claims; and whether it is possible for evidence-based medicine to truly be value free. The final chapter argues that the most important question we can ask is not, "How can we separate values from science?" but, "In a democratic society, how can we decide in a politically and morally acceptable way what values should drive science?"

Key features:

- introduces complex philosophical issues in a manner accessible to non-professional academics;
- critically examines philosophical assumptions made in medicine, providing a better understanding of medicine that can lead to better healthcare;
- integrates medical examples and historic contexts so as to frame the rationale of philosophical views and provide lively illustrations of how philosophy can impact science and our lives;
- uses interconnected chapters to demonstrate that disparate philosophical concepts are deeply related (e.g., it shows how the aims of medicine inform how we should understand theoretical reasoning).

Dien Ho is an Associate Professor of Philosophy and Healthcare Ethics at MCPHS University, USA. His recent publications include an edited anthology, *Philosophical Issues in Pharmaceutics: Development, Dispensing, and Use* (2017). He has also written for non-academic publications including *Newsweek*, *Philosophy Now!*, *The Boston Globe*, and other popular media.

A PHILOSOPHER GOES TO THE DOCTOR

A Critical Look at Philosophical Assumptions in Medicine

Dien Ho

Routledge
Taylor & Francis Group
NEW YORK AND LONDON

First published 2019
by Routledge
52 Vanderbilt Avenue, New York, NY 10017

and by Routledge
2 Park Square, Milton Park, Abingdon, Oxon, OX14 4RN

Routledge is an imprint of the Taylor & Francis Group, an informa business

Library of Congress Cataloging-in-Publication Data
A catalog record for this title has been requested

ISBN: 978-1-138-64778-7 (hbk)
ISBN: 978-1-138-64779-4 (pbk)
ISBN: 978-1-315-62687-1 (ebk)

Typeset in Bembo
by Apex CoVantage, LLC

CONTENTS

ANNOTATED TABLE OF CONTENTS

of bemoaning the ineliminable presence of values, we examine arguments offered by philosophers so that we can collectively decide what kind of values we want in science. Ultimately, the important question is not how we can make science value-free but, as a liberal democratic society, how can we decide in a politically and morally acceptable way what values should drive science.

Dedication

Dedications are usually not elaborate and overly personal, but I think I'll break that rule. My mother was born in China shortly before the onset of the Second Sino-Japanese War. She recounted stories of emerging from air raid shelters as a child only to see the bodies of unfortunate neighbors who didn't manage to seek safety fast enough. After the war, economic opportunities brought her and her family to Taiwan where she lived until the end of her high school days. Graduating first in her class at a prestigious girls' school, she was chosen to represent all high school students in a meeting with Chiang Kai-shek. Her parents discouraged her from studying overseas, but witnessing her friends' departures to colleges and universities around the world was too much for her. So, she borrowed money from her high school teachers and applied to and was accepted by two colleges: Sarah Lawrence College in New York and Talladega College in Alabama. She chose Talladega—a historically black university founded by freed slaves. Living in the Jim Crow South was eye-opening. I asked her once if she used the "colored" or "white" facilities. She replied that she always just did whatever she wanted because no one quite knew how their bifurcated bigotry would apply to a young Chinese woman. "I might as well have been a Martian," she would say.

During summers, she traveled to Atlantic City where she worked as a life-guard during the day, a waitress at night, and a cocktail waitress afterwards. Those gigs were her only means of making enough money to sustain herself through college. My father was sketching portraits on the boardwalk when they met. She had always remarked on how terrible his portraits were and how no one would pay for them upon completion.

My father was a student at Williams College in Massachusetts and, in his infinite charm, convinced my mother to transfer to Williams. At the time, Williams was an all-male school. My mother enrolled as a special student while working as an au pair for the dean. I have tried to look for records of her matriculation there, but Williams has none, likely because her circumstances were so unique. Other than a photograph of their wedding in the courtyard of Dean Brooks' home, there is no evidence of her presence.

While my dad pursued his graduate degree in architecture, my mother was accepted into a program in landscape architecture at Harvard University. But her pregnancy with my oldest sister suspended her study plans. During her final days, she showed me the acceptance letter and asked if they would still honor it.

My parents returned to Hong Kong in 1964, where my father's parents lived. There, he started a successful architectural business. My mother's interests and background in fine arts led her to open the first graphic art gallery in Hong Kong specializing in Western art. The two of them were in the cultural vanguard, playing hosts to visiting scholars, artists, and intellectuals. Among the cassette tapes I found in my mother's belongings was one labeled "Bucky Fuller's dinner lecture." He had apparently come to our home for dinner and gave an impromptu talk on the future of architecture. As some of their friends have remarked to me, they were a breath of fresh air in a hyper capitalistic system.

After a bitter divorce, she secured the custody of her three children but was financially bereft. She struggled mightily to eke out a living in Hong Kong—a city where she had no family and whose language was foreign to her—supported only by the few friends who did not align themselves with my more famous father. She sold Chinese paintings to wealthy clients to buy my violin—a fact she often reminded me of, especially when I didn't practice. After 20 or so years of struggle, she managed to secure our immigration to the United States. Her reasons for leaving Hong Kong were complex. Along with her desire to find solace in a place away from my father who was frequently trying to regain custody of his children, she also knew that we would fail miserably in the rigid education system of Hong Kong.

As a teenager, I would engage in days-long arguments with my mother over intellectual issues. I would proclaim that all modern art is garbage, created to fool us into agreeing to its merits and worth. She would bring me to Boston's Museum of Fine Arts and schooled me in the texture of paint, the play on space, and the meta-philosophy of an artist. These conversations sparked my interests in philosophy. She convinced me that debating intellectual matters was fun and important.

While I was finishing my dissertation as a newlywed living in Tennessee, I received a phone call from her. She might have stomach cancer. Earlier in the summer, I had taken her to an emergency room because she was unable to swallow any fluid for days. Her reluctance to seek medical care had a great deal to do with the fact that she was too poor to afford health insurance. I paid for the visit with half of my graduate stipend and she promised to go for a follow-up visit, but she never did. For a woman who never smoked, rarely drank, ate a pristine diet, and ran long distance, I was convinced that the oncologist had made a terrible mistake and that a weekend visit to Boston would clear up the matter.

As I pulled up to the house in late afternoon, it was already dark. I saw a thin figure on the front lawn raking leaves. It was my mother. As I hugged her, I realized how small she had gotten. The obstruction in her gastro-esophagus junction had made it impossible for her to eat properly. I chastised her for being out raking leaves. She protested: Her son was coming home. How could she leave a mess of leaves strewn all over the front lawn?

Nine months after the initial diagnosis, she passed away. She died at the exact median life-expectancy of a person with stage-IV gastric cancer. She was 63 years old. During the demanding two rounds of chemotherapy, she vomited, lost her hair, and forced herself to eat. But, at no point did she remark on the unfairness of the turn of events. For the first time in her life, she owned a house and she was working as a tai-chi instructor at a neighboring college. There was stability. After the CT scans showed that the second round of chemo had made no significant difference, I could not uphold the façade of bravery, broke down, and cried on her chest. She was the one who comforted me: "You silly boy. You have taken care of me so well. I hope you will have a child who will take care of you as well as you have taken care of me."

However meager my intellectual accomplishments, none would have been possible had my mother not taken remarkable risks and made tremendous sacrifices for the betterment of her children. Beyond her care and affection for arts and letters, it was her fearlessness that I admire. She trusted herself, and her confidence brought us all a sense of comfort when the world literally changed around us.

It is to my late mother Chi-Ping Lu that I dedicate this book. May you be proud of who I am.

A NOTE ON THE COVER

The painting "Dulce et Decorum Est" depicts the chemical structure of Cytoxan—a chemotherapy agent that saved my friend and the artist Bonnie Ashmore's life. The work's title comes from a WWI poem by Wilfred Owen on the devastating effects of mustard gas used on soldiers. Two decades later, on the eve of WWII, while researching an antidote for mustard gas, Dr. Louis Goodman and Dr. Alfred Gilman of Yale University combed through medical records of soldiers exposed to mustard gas in WWI. What they found was remarkable: many of the survivors had lower counts of white blood cells. Goodman and Gilman hypothesized that whatever property in mustard gas that destroyed white blood cells could also be used to fight mutated immune cells in cancer patients. Their theory proved correct, and nitrogen mustard molecules became the basis of Cytoxan—an effective treatment for lymphomas, brain cancer, leukemia, and other solid tumors.

Bonnie Ashmore is a painter and printmaker who holds an MFA from American University. She completed her undergraduate studies at Brandeis University, where she received a BA in Fine Arts and a Post-Baccalaureate Certificate in Painting. Bonnie has been a practicing artist and educator for nearly 2 decades and is full-time faculty at North Shore Community College in the Fine Arts/Visual Studies Department. She is a member of Gallery 263 in Cambridge, MA and has shown her work in many group and solo shows in New England, New York, Washington DC, Maryland, Florida, and Nova Scotia, Canada. Her work has been reviewed by Howard Halle, juried by Jerry Saltz, and is held in many private collections. To learn more about Bonnie and her work, please visit: www.bonnieashmore.com.

INTRODUCTION

Quackery is a bad thing. No one goes to a party and proudly proclaims he is a quack by trade. What makes quackery bad, among other things, is that it provides no therapeutic benefits or that it might harm patients. Yet many conventional medical therapies are harmful and provide marginal benefits, if any. Consider vertebroplasty—a common out-patient procedure that injects cement into a patient's vertebrae to fill fractures and relieve pain. The procedure is performed hundreds of thousands of times annually all over the United States. In 2009, Medicaid paid $2,000 each for 40,000 procedures performed that year (Langreth, 2009). But two randomized studies, including one by Firanescu et al. (2018), showed that vertebroplasties yield results no better than their sham counterparts in which no insertion is made and no cement injected.[1] Still, vertebroplasties remain the standard treatment for back fractures.

Similarly, in a meta-analysis involving 718 patients, Fournier et al. (2010) concluded that selective serotonin re-uptake inhibitors (SSRIs) did not meaningfully improve the symptoms of patients suffering from mild to moderate depression compared to placebos. The study has been cited over 1,730 times since its publication; nevertheless, SSRIs continue to be prescribed as the first-line pharmacological treatment for depression. If the lack of therapeutic benefits is the hallmark of quackery, then many conventional medical practices would seem to qualify as quackery.

It is also not bad intent that makes something quackery. Lots of quacks sincerely believe they are providing effective care. And physicians do not always have their patients' best interests in mind. Defensive medicine leads to the prescribing of tests and treatments that are of marginal use simply because physicians want to minimize possible legal exposure. In a 2014 study of three Massachusetts hospitals, Rothberg et al. (2014) concluded that 28% of services ordered were wholly or partly based on defensive medicine. There are of course more innocent examples as well. Clinicians sometimes write a script for prescription-strength pain medications, like ibuprofen, or recommend vitamins just so their patients can feel like they are taking something to help their woes and leave the doctor's office satisfied. Acting so out of self-interest cannot be the distinguishing mark of quackery, for many physicians do that as well. What, then, is the difference between being a self-serving clinician and being a quack? Quackery is bad presumably because it is not *real* medicine. Even if someone swears up and down that a recent visit to a faith healer has rid him of his plantar fasciitis, the improvement, we instinctively think, is luck at best or is "all in his head." Given enough time, he will go see a real doctor. Modern medicine represents not only our best means of maintaining and improving our health; we trust it because it is grounded in science, evidence, and theories that are consistent with our broader scientific worldview. Science is often seen as the epitome of how to pursue knowledge. Need a little more cachet and respectability for one's discipline and practice? Add "science" to the title (e.g., political science), sprinkle some scientific-sounding methodologies and jargon into one's research, wear a white lab coat on TV, and create journals and accreditation agencies complete with peer review and assessments.

Modern medicine is great because it works and it is based on science. Yet, as straightforward a defense of medicine as it seems, a curious soul might have the nagging feeling that the specialness of medicine is not so obvious. For starters, if medicine is science-based, one naturally wonders what exactly makes something a *science*. Known to philosophers as the demarcation problem, it has proven to be an exceedingly difficult question to answer. Medicine has certainly improved our lives, but is it because of the science of medicine or something completely different?[2] After all, quackery could work too but we wouldn't call it scientific medicine. And, of course, when we say that medicine works, we need to know what exactly is meant by "works." Has medicine made our lives better? If we measure it in terms of longevity, this might be true (assuming that the credit goes to medicine). But what is the price we pay to get there? Are there "externalities" (think of our water supply that is tainted with pharmacological run-offs) that we are unaware of, such that once we have added up the costs and the benefits of modern medicine, we are actually in the red? Here, philosophers can earn their paychecks and help answer these questions. The aim of this book is to look at the philosophical concepts at the basis of modern medicine in a way that is accessible to non-philosophers. Practitioners in research and clinical medicine are often entirely unaware that they are making philosophical assumptions that are critical to their disciplines. Understanding what makes for sound medicine can improve how we do research and how we provide clinical care. It is this grand wish to improve the practice of medicine that drives this book.

In Chapter 1, we examine the alleged line between science and pseudoscience. The post-positivist philosopher Karl Popper famously suggested in the 1950s that the difference lies in science's ability to generate falsifiable predictions.

The idea is that unless one's discipline can create predictions that *can* be false, one is not practicing science. Although most contemporary philosophers have long rejected Popper's view, falsifiability continues to dominate academic discussion and education in medicine. Indeed, one of my earliest moments of realizing something was amiss in medicine came at a conference where a prominent geneticist said that since what he was doing was not falsifiable, he did not consider himself a scientist. I thought to myself, "Well, if you aren't a scientist, then no one here is." The dogma of falsifiability badly needs to be shattered. Knowing if and where the distinction between science and pseudo-science lies can help us mark out the boundary of scientific medicine. Therapeutic options, grants for research, and even the methods of how we study the human body would all be affected by the outcome of this discussion.

In Chapter 2, we explore the main attempts to define health as well as diseases and disabilities. The emergence of the autism-rights movement highlights some of the tricky issues. Specifically, is autism a disorder in search of a cure or is it a form of "neurodiversity," as proponents of autism rights suggest? Drawing on the Civil Rights Movement, autism-rights advocates argue that we should find ways to ensure that autists are not unfairly discriminated against in a neurotypical society. How we understand what constitutes health has a profound impact on resource allocation, clinical medicine, and what research goals we ought to pursue. More importantly, our concept of what makes for a healthy person also tells us a great deal about what we are fundamentally from a physiological point of view.

Chapters 3, 4, and 5 are inter-related and they examine the concept of evidence, which is clearly important to science. One might even suggest that the demand for empirical support for one's claim is what distinguishes science from other disciplines. In the past few decades, Evidence-Based Medicine has been become an industry standard (in name, if not in spirit). Starting with the work of 18th century Scottish philosopher David Hume, philosophers have realized that evidence and how it supports a hypothesis are hardly transparent matters. If we don't understand what constitutes evidence (and how different types offer different support), it would be premature to commit wholesale to, say, the epistemic virtues of randomized clinical trials.

One typical way clinicians diagnose patients is to infer the diagnoses that best explain their patients' symptoms. Dry cough, fever, tiny white spots around reddish areas, the lack of MMR vaccination, and exposure to patients who have been diagnosed with measles: these all point to an obvious culprit—the patient has contracted measles. Inferring a hypothesis on the basis of its ability to explain the evidence at hand is both a common and valuable method of logical reasoning. Philosophers, however, have realized that this method of reasoning faces numerous formidable challenges. For starters, plenty of false theories (e.g., Newtonian mechanics) can explain certain observations; the connection between explanatory power and truth seems more tenuous than we believe. In Chapter 4, we look at some of the most common theories of explanation. Not only would this help us understand, as a mode of reasoning, how inference to the best explanation (IBE) works; it will also tell us whether science and medicine should care about searching for explanations. Perhaps science can do just fine without knowing *why* things happen.

It seems clear that a good piece of evidence should increase the probability that a hypothesis (which it aims to support) is true. In this sense, to understand the concept of evidence, we need to know what we mean by probability. Moreover, since medicine, like most empirical sciences, makes probabilistic claims, we ought to have a clear grasp of what it means when, say, we learn that a treatment has an 82% chance of success. Is it a measurement of the clinician's confidence? If so, is there an objective measure as to whether her assessment is correct? If it is a breakdown of some clinical trials (e.g., 82 out of 100 subjects responded well to the treatment), how does that number affect *me*? Probabilistic claims are everywhere in the uncertain world of medicine; for researchers, clinicians, and patients, it behooves us to learn about the challenges and complexities of different interpretations of probability.

The final two chapters focus on the role of values in clinical and research medicine. While the physician-patient relationship has pivoted away from medical paternalism towards emphasizing the patient's autonomy, many have assumed that value-free medicine is both possible and desirable. It is widely accepted in linguistics and the philosophy of language that everyday communication requires that we make some basic assumptions about our values. "Another round of drinks for everyone" does not mean everyone on the face of the planet. A bartender who assumes that his generous customer is intent on treating all of humanity to a free beverage will have a long night and a short career in bartending. More importantly, the very nature of logical reasoning—something that is seemingly devoid of any subjectivity—depends a great deal on our personal values. Given the fact that there are many logical systems, the choice of which one to use must be based on "extra-logical" considerations, such as expediency, simplicity, and usefulness. Rationality and epistemology are both deeply value-laden and, as such, any social activities that involve them are also necessarily value-laden. If clinical medicine cannot be value-free, the question becomes what sort of values should guide our practice instead.

One of the grand dreams of logical positivism—an intellectual movement that dominated the first half of the 20th century—is that however biased, wishful, or self-interested a researcher is, the logical method of science is immune to these social and psychological influences. Science, like justice, is supposedly blind. The Great Firewall between the context of science and the inner-working of science has been crumbling since the 1960s. In the final chapter, we look at arguments by Helen Longino and Kathleen Okruhlik that aim to show that values are ineliminable in science. But rather than surrendering to relativism or radical subjectivism, we can take the reins. We can shape the direction and methodology of research medicine in a manner akin to other value-laden social institutions, like public education, politics, and urban planning. Our ability to maneuver and come together in a community filled with diverse values can teach us important lessons of how we can do so in medicine. Welcome to the real world, so to speak.

The purpose of this book is not to look at modern medicine with deep skepticism. Although many of the philosophical problems remained unsolved, that doesn't mean we should abandon medicine. Lack of justification for certain beliefs and practices only means we should dial back our confidence and certainty. Perhaps through humility, a better medicine will emerge.

The writing of this book could not have been possible had it not been for the help and support of many people. My wonderful colleagues in the School of Arts and Sciences at MCPHS University (formerly, Massachusetts College of Pharmacy and Health Sciences) provided invaluable insights. Joe DeMasi, Roger Denome, Crystal Ellis, Martha Gardner, Frances Keech, Magdalena Luca, and Ken Richman came to my rescue when I needed help with genetics, biology, history of medicine, radiography, statistics, and philosophy of medicine. It is a joy to be a part of such a supportive and knowledgeable faculty. My assistants Mandy Smith and Amy Pak provided crucial feedback and logistical support. My long-time friends and philosophy colleagues Bradley Monton and Michael Ridge expertly commented on early drafts; the book improved because of them. Project Manager Autumn Spalding's sharp eyes, remarkable patience, and hard work transformed the final production process from a mad dash to the finish line into a swan's glide across a tranquil lake in Switzerland. The bulk of the writing process took place at Forge Baking Company in Somerville, Massachusetts, a perfect spot for me. Thanks to the staff who welcomed my prolonged occupation. Finally, to my editor and father-in-law Peter Leo, who pounced on unclear prose and grammatical errors, all the while admonishing the author to make the book accessible to non-academic readers—I hope I have succeeded. And, of course, I am grateful for his daughter, my wife Jane, who indulged my unbridled enthusiasm when I felt the need to share some fantastic tale from medicine regardless of the time of day. She has my love and admiration.

Notes

1 Sham vertebroplasties present a particularly interesting example of the power of placebo treatments. Unlike the use of placeboes to treat "subjectivity heavy" conditions such as irritable bowel syndrome or arthritic pain where presumably placeboes treatments can "rewire" the brain to lessen the discomfort, vertebroplasties involve skeletal injuries. For an excellent look at the research on placeboes, follow Ted Kaptchuk's work. For instance, in an on-going study led by Sarah Ballou (with the participation of Kaptchuk), they look to confirm results (from prior studies) that placeboes can provide significant therapeutic benefits even if patients know they are taking placeboes (2017).

2 Many cultures have traditional folk remedies and some of them are therapeutically beneficial. Presumably, their success is independent of their scientific status.

References

Ballou, S., Kaptchuk, T. J., Hirsch, W., Nee, J., Iturrino, J., Hall, K. T., . . . Davis, R. B. (2017). Open-label versus double-blind placebo treatment in irritable bowel syndrome: Study protocol for a randomized controlled trial. *Trials*, *18*(1), 234. doi:10.1186/s13063-017-1964-x

Firanescu, C. E., de Vries, J., Lodder, P., Venmans, A., Schoemaker, M. C., Smeet, A. J., . . . Lohle, P. N. M. (2018). Vertebroplasty versus sham procedure for painful acute osteoporotic vertebral compression fractures (VERTOS IV): Randomised sham controlled clinical trial. *BMJ: British Medical Journal, 361.* doi:10.1136/bmj.k1551

Fournier, J. C., DeRubeis, R. J., Hollon, S. D., Dimidjian, S., Amsterdam, J. D., Shelton, R. C., & Fawcett, J. (2010). Antidepressant drug effects and depression severity: A patient-level meta-analysis. *JAMA: The Journal of the American Medical Association, 303*(1), 47–53. doi:10.1001/jama.2009.1943

Langreth, R. (2009). Common spine surgery shows no benefit. *Forbes.*

Rothberg, M. B., Class, J., Bishop, T. F., Friderici, J., Kleppel, R., & Lindenauer, P. K. (2014). The cost of defensive medicine on 3 hospital medicine services. *JAMA Internal Medicine, 174*(11), 1867–1868. doi:10.1001/jamainternmed.2014.4649

1

THE BOUNDARIES OF MEDICINE

1.1 What If Spooky Stuff Works?

One of the main goals of medicine is to improve the health of individuals. This much, it seems, is indisputable. But what exactly constitutes medicine? There are many ways to improve someone's health. A 2012 study suggests that individuals who obtain college degrees after the age of 25 have lower risks for depression and better self-rated health (Walsemann, Bell, & Hummer, 2012). Although completing a college degree seems to be correlated with better health, it would be odd for a physician to recommend that patients enroll in a college or university to stave off mid-life depression. The reason is not the lack of a robust causal connection between education and health. For a doctor to recommend higher education as a prophylactic against depression seems professionally inappropriate.[1] We want physicians to practice medicine. Just because something improves your health, it doesn't follow that it falls within the domain of medicine.

Or does it?

The issue is not merely a question of how medicine should delimit its professional identity; for example, defining the sorts of skills a doctor should have. Where we draw the boundaries of medicine can have substantive effects on the quality of life for millions of people. Must we wait until adequate evidence from randomized clinical trials (the gold standard for experimental science) emerges before we permit public access to the treatments? Should we allocate resources to provide alternative treatments that fall outside of mainstream medicine? Should prayers be encouraged in a hospital if clinical trials show that patients' outcomes improve after praying? Can bad science or non-science be good medicine?

Modern Western medicine prides itself on being based on science. In their essay "Engineers, Cranks, Physicians, Magicians," published in *The New England Journal of Medicine*, Clark Glymour and Douglas Stalker say:

> Medicine in industrialized nations is scientific medicine. The claim tacitly made by American or European physicians, and tacitly relied on by their patients, is that their palliatives and procedures have been shown by science to be effective. Although the physician's medical practice is not itself science, it is based on science and on training that is supposed to teach physicians to apply scientific knowledge to people in a rational way.
>
> *(1983, p. 960)*

Treatment protocols are not merely bits of wisdom passed from generation to generation of healers. They are grounded in a rich scientific underpinning that helps form a coherent picture of how our bodies work. A conflict between a potential therapy and well-accepted scientific beliefs automatically raises doubts about the efficacy of the therapy. If AIDS patients who were prayed for, unbeknownst to them, by faraway strangers have fewer AIDS-related diseases when compared to the control group (Sicher, Targ, Moore, & Smith, 1998), we tend

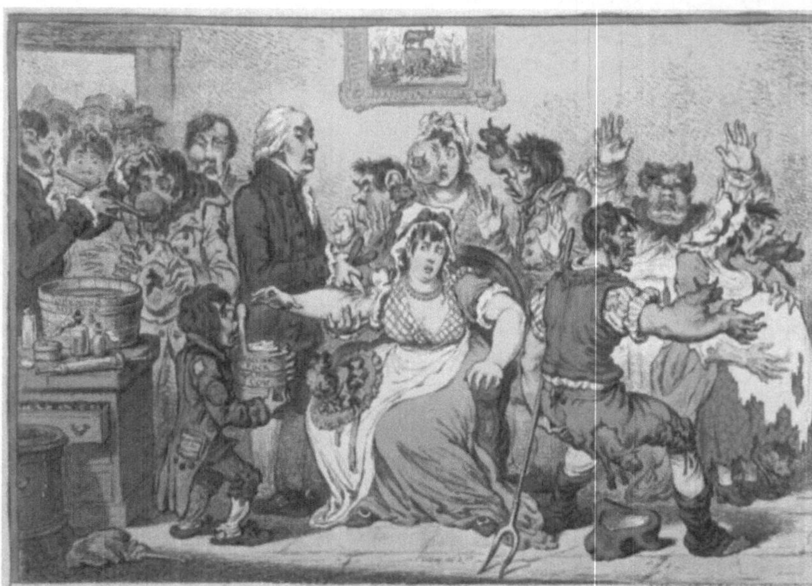
The Cow Pock — or — the Wonderful Effects of the New Inoculation! —

FIGURE 1.1 The Cow Pock

Source: The British satirist James Gillray's rendition of the Smallpox and Inoculation Hospital at St. Pancras (1802). Miniature cows emerge from the sites of cowpox incisions.

to conclude that the results are clinical outliers or that there must be some unidentified naturalistic process that further investigation would discover. Not only is this a reasonable reaction in medicine, it is what any proponent of the modern scientific worldview would do when she observes something seemingly miraculous. To subscribe to a scientific understanding of the world requires at a minimum a rejection of "spooky explanations"—supernatural explanations (e.g., non-physical divine interventions) that conflict with widely accepted scientific beliefs.

Of course, defining what is "spooky" is a tricky matter. The history of science is filled with episodes where once paradoxical or spooky results eventually gain enough converts to become mainstream science. Edward Jenner's discovery and subsequent advocacy of using cowpox to vaccinate against smallpox was met with resistance not only from the clergy on the charge that it was unnatural but also from the medical and scientific community at large. Furthermore, if we define "spooky" as something that is not explicable using the language of science alone, then we risk turning the claim that science rejects spooky explanations into the trivial truth that science rejects explanations that science rejects.

Nevertheless, if we think that medical practices from clinical to research settings ought to be grounded in science (treatment recommendations should be supported by scientific evidence, for instance), then it follows that what is not science is automatically not medicine. Indeed, a common justification for the uniqueness or privileged status of modern medicine is that it is science-based. The distinction between science and non-science thus becomes a relevant matter for medicine: to identify the boundaries of modern scientific medicine requires delineating the boundaries of science.

1.2 Verificationism: From Metaphysics to Pseudo-science

The modern discussion of where we ought to draw the line between science and non-science arguably began with the works of the logical positivists of Vienna and Berlin in the 1920s. From the start of the 20th century, Europe witnessed an explosion in scientific advances. From Albert Einstein's remarkable theory that light behaves both as particles and as waves (1905) to Chadwick's discovery of neutrons (1932), from Landsteiner's identification of blood types (1900) to Fleming's introduction of penicillin (1929), the first half of 20th century was a time of incredible scientific advances that revolutionized the way we understand the world and ourselves.

Impressed by the progress in empirical science, the positivists strived to model other intellectual endeavors (principally, philosophy) in the same mold. To do so, of course, they would need to identify what distinguishes science from other ways of understanding the world. What makes the new empirical science of the 20th century so incredibly successful? Is it possible for philosophy and other intellectual endeavors to adopt this methodology?

It is important to appreciate the historical context of the positivists. The first half of the 20th century was a tumultuous time in Europe. Along with the dazzling advances in mathematics and the empirical sciences, Europe was undergoing a series of cultural and political upheavals. The mechanical efficiency of a brutal world war driven by old-world political fissures, the devastating Spanish Influenza that killed 20–40 million people worldwide, the Great Depression, the rise of fascism, ethnic cleansings on an unfathomable scale, and a deadlier and more widespread world war culminating in the dropping of two atomic bombs—all of these highlighted the power of modern science and the grave consequences of ignorance, bigotry, and tribalism.[2]

From a philosophical point of view, at the turn of the 20th century, post-Kantian idealism was still the dominant school of thought in continental Europe. Like any broad philosophical movement, variations of idealism run a wide gamut; however, one of its central tenets is that we have no access to the world in and of itself. The nature of reality instead depends on how we think about it; that is, questions of ontology (what exists) and how things interact with one another can only be asked and settled relative to a particular way of conceptualizing the world. Since there is no objective reality to adjudicate between competing theories of the world, disagreements about the nature of the world become detached from objective empirical feedbacks. In other words, between two competing metaphysical views of the world (e.g., do possible objects exist?), no amount of empirical evidence could settle the disagreement. At a time when philosophy and science, especially physics, were still academically intertwined, the tremendous advances made by modern physics must have made speculative and empirically empty philosophizing of this sort less than compelling. The positivist project was first and foremost an attempt to borrow the blueprint of empirical science to rebuild the philosophical house.

The success of science, the positivists noticed, was ultimately rooted in the centrality of empirical content. Specifically, scientific statements are those that can be empirically tested or verified. To be sure, there was much disagreement in terms of what exactly constituted verification, e.g., do these statements need to be actually verified or do they only need to be verifiable in principle? What exactly does "in principle" mean? What constitutes verification? These are serious problems that forced the positivists to frequently modify their definition of empirical verifiability. Indeed, some of these nagging problems that initially seemed to be minor technical obstacles would eventually reveal devastating flaws in the positivist project. Nevertheless, defining science as rooted in empirical verification held much promise, especially against the backdrop of speculative metaphysics of the 19th century. In essence, a statement is scientific if it has empirical consequences; e.g., it entails empirical observations that can be measured, tested, confirmed, refuted, and so on.

The power of the positivist's verificationism might seem subtle at first sight, but its epistemic implications are staggering. Take, for instance, the verifiability criterion of meaning that was favored by British positivist A.J. Ayer. The idea is that a sentence has meaning only insofar as it can be empirically confirmed or refuted. A speculative claim about the nature of reality that is immune to empirical testing is literally meaningless.[3] Two theories that have the same verification processes are, according to this criterion, synonymous. Empirically empty disagreements among philosophers turned out to be no more than empty disagreements about meaningless statements. In one fell swoop, the positivists seemingly undercut much of orthodox philosophy while capturing exactly what makes modern science so special.

The positivists were certainly not the first philosophers who advocated a kind of empirical housecleaning. In section XII of his *An Inquiry Concerning Human Understanding*, the great 18th century Scottish philosopher David Hume famously suggests that, for any work, we must ask, "[D]oes it contain any abstract reasoning concerning quantity or number? No. Does it contain any experimental reasoning concerning matter of fact or existence? No. Commit it then to the flames, for it can be nothing but sophistry and illusion." Likewise, echoing Hume's view, Ernst Mach—another pioneer of positivist ideas—remarks that "[w]here neither confirmation nor refutation is possible, science is not concerned. Science acts and acts only in the domain of *uncompleted* experience" (Mach, 1988, p. 587, emphasis in original).

The emergence of empirical verification as the defining characteristic of modern science also provided philosophers with a ready tool to delineate science from pseudo-science. Although all pseudo-sciences are, by definition, not sciences, it is not true that all non-sciences are pseudo-sciences. Predicting one's future using tarot cards is not a science in any straightforward sense, but it also does not pretend to be one. To be a pseudo-science, a discipline must attempt to be a science while failing to be so. Along with the emergence of the impressive breakthroughs in early 20th century science, there were also disciplines and theories that assumed the appearance of science without actually being science (at least according to positivists). Practices and studies like zone therapies (an early form of reflexology), phrenology (determining personalities and mental acuity by measuring the size and shape of someone's skull), and spiritual evolution (a marriage of spiritualism and bits and pieces of Darwinian evolution) also flourished.[4]

Verificationism seems like a perfect way to separate genuine sciences from the pretenders. Modern physics, for instance, makes empirical predictions. If Planck's idea that high-energy particles come in discrete units of energy is correct, we should be able to build a device (e.g., a Geiger counter) to measure radiation that would give us discrete readings. More radiation should lead to more discrete "clicks" (as opposed to a continuum of non-discrete signals like gradually increasing volume). On the other hand, pseudo-sciences appear to lack the same level of empirical implication. When a person dies and a spiritualist posits that the soul departs the body, how are we to measure that? Do we use a scale? Do souls have weight? Souls might exist, but unless there is a way to manipulate them, measure them, and observe their effects, they are causally inert. The positivists' verificationism tells us that, without entailing empirical observations, statements about souls are not scientific claims.

1.3 The End of Verificationism

As intuitively plausible as verificationism appeared, many positivists saw immediately the difficulties with it as a way to distinguish science from non-science. For starters, universal statements such as "All metals expand when heated" cannot be verified by any *finite* set of empirical observations. The "scope" (what the statement is *about*) of a universal claim is infinitely large, and no amount of confirmation can exhaustively verify it. But there is also a more practical problem: verificationism seems to be both too loose and too strict as a demarcation criterion between science and pseudo-science. Let's return to the spiritualism example. The proponents of spiritualism only have to posit that souls have weight in order to turn what appears to be pseudo-science into science. A Massachusetts doctor, Duncan MacDougall (1866–1920), attempted to measure the weight of souls. He

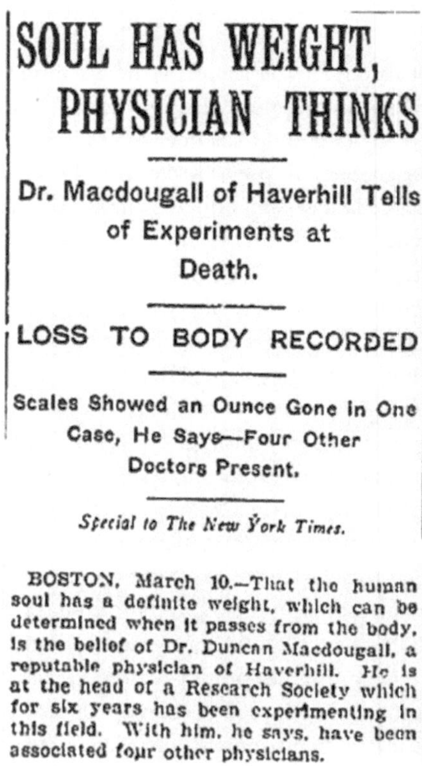

SOUL HAS WEIGHT, PHYSICIAN THINKS

Dr. Macdougall of Haverhill Tells of Experiments at Death.

LOSS TO BODY RECORDED

Scales Showed an Ounce Gone in One Case, He Says—Four Other Doctors Present.

Special to The New York Times.

BOSTON, March 10.—That the human soul has a definite weight, which can be determined when it passes from the body, is the belief of Dr. Duncan Macdougall, a reputable physician of Haverhill. He is at the head of a Research Society which for six years has been experimenting in this field. With him, he says, have been associated four other physicians.

FIGURE 1.2 MacDougall's Experiment

Source: New York Times' frontpage headline from March 10, 1907 on MacDougall's experiment.

weighed six tuberculosis patients before and after they died. He concluded that the difference of three-fourths of an ounce must have been the weights of the souls. He also measured a number of dogs and detected no weight differences; thus, according to MacDougall, dogs have no souls. Verificationism would consider Dr. MacDougall's project as perfectly scientific.

Of course, the spiritualist theory that souls exist and have weight might be false, but there is a big difference between being a false theory and being a pseudo-scientific theory. We now know that Newtonian mechanics is false; mass, for instance, is not conserved in a closed system (per Einstein's groundbreaking discovery). But Newtonian mechanics is still science, albeit false science. Similarly, until German virologist Harald zur Hausen demonstrated the connection between HPV and cervical cancer in the early 1980s, mainstream oncology rejected the claim that cancer could be caused by viruses. Oncologists were wrong about the link between viruses and cancer prior to this discovery, but it did not render past oncology a pseudo-science. The truth of a theory, in this sense, is independent of its scientific status. If what is required of a science is that it entails some empirical results, then verificationism risks making it too easy for any discipline to qualify as a science.

In addition to being too permissive, verificationism would also deny the scientific status of many accepted sciences on the ground that they do not entail any empirical implications. Formal sciences like computation theory cannot be confirmed or refuted with empirical methods. Observational sciences that aim to collect data do not necessarily involve the testing of hypotheses. A team of scientists, for example, that measures ocean temperatures at various depths and offers no empirical hypotheses would not be doing science according to verificationism (since there is no hypothesis to verify or to test). The same problem applies to other more theoretical sciences, from theoretical physics to sub-fields in system research and in formal linguistics.

1.4 Karl Popper's Falsifiability

In light of the difficulty verificationism faced, the British-Austrian philosopher Karl Popper proposed an alternative demarcation between science and pseudo-science. Popper's critique of the positivists' verificationism centers around his argument against induction as a scientific method. Inductive reasoning takes limited observed samples and makes projections of things that we have not observed. A simple example might look something like this: we have observed 5,421,977 emeralds and every one of them has been green, and we have not observed any non-green emeralds; therefore, we infer that the next emerald will likely be green or that all emeralds in the universe are in fact green. Inductive inferences in medicine are common. For instance, if we have observed that all the patients who suffered from general paresis also had untreated late-stage syphilis, we might infer that, as a general rule, one can only develop paresis as a result of untreated late-stage syphilis. Unlike deductive inferences (such as classical logic or Euclidean geometry), the conclusions of inductive arguments are never guaranteed by the truth of the premises; they are only made more or less plausible relative to the observed samples. As we learn in college statistics courses, the strength of an inductive inference depends on two factors: the size of our sample and whether our sample is biased.

Consider the sample size criterion for a moment. Suppose I want to know what percentage of U.S. voters are smokers. Suppose that there are 146 million registered voters. If I were to poll a dozen voters to see how many of them smoke, the confidence I have in my projection would be fairly low. We can think of our confidence as a ratio of the number of voters I polled (n) divided by the number of voters (m). As n/m approaches 1, our confidence in our projection increases; that is, as I poll more people, my confidence goes up. Empirical sciences rely on this sort of inductive reasoning. It allows us to make justified claims about things that we have not observed on the basis of observed evidence. We believe that smoking causes cancer because we have observed higher rates of cancer among smokers than among non-smokers.[5] Indeed, the positivists' idea of empirical confirmation can largely be understood as an exercise in inductive reasoning. A scientific theory, according to the positivists, makes empirical predictions about events that we have not observed. When one does an experiment and obtains results that were predicted by the theory, we say that the theory is confirmed by the experimental results.

Popper's argument against inductive reasoning focuses on the idea that most scientific claims are universal in character; that is, they are about *all* possible observations entailed by the claims. For instance, the claim "All metals expand when heated" concerns not just actual pieces of metal. It also ranges over past pieces of metal that we have not observed and future pieces of metal. The claim tells us, for instance, that if we find metal on Alpha Centauri, we are confident that it would expand when heated. Moreover, we can even make inferences about hypothetical pieces of metal as well. If Lady Macbeth's dagger were made out of metal, it would expand when heated. We believe these claims are true because *all* metals expand when heated. The word "all" ranges over not only actual metals but over past, future, and hypothetical metals as well. Similarly, we can say the same thing about many other universal empirical claims; e.g., had Lady Macbeth smoked cigarettes, she would have had an elevated risk for certain types of cancer.

Given the universal nature of many scientific claims, and given the fact that we measure the strength of an inductive inference as a ratio between the observed sample and the total range of our claim (i.e., n/m), Popper concludes that no universal scientific claim can be confirmed. The range (m) of a universal claim is

TABLE 1.1 The relationship between sample size and confidence in an inductive conclusion

n/m = our confidence in the conclusion of an inductive inference (in terms of sample size)	n = the size of our sample m = the size of the conclusion or projection

infinitely large (since "all" ranges over an infinite number of objects); therefore, no matter how large our sample is (n), we will always have zero confidence in our projection! Worse yet, additional experimental observations will not increase our confidence in our inference, since no matter how many more experiments we perform, n will always be a finite number. The ratio of $(n + 1)/m$ where m is infinite in size will always remain 0.

In a 1953 lecture at Peterhouse College of Cambridge University, Popper elaborated on his critique of verificationism and proposed a new way of demarcating science from pseudo-science. Popper notes that many pseudo-sciences have

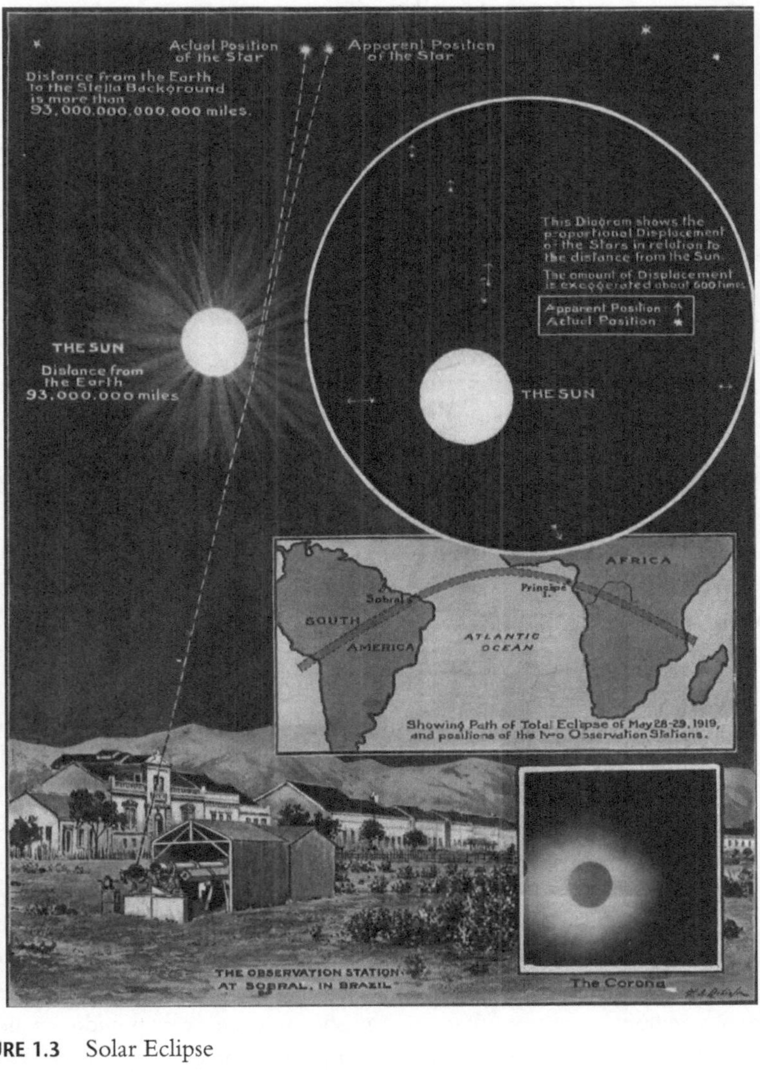

FIGURE 1.3 Solar Eclipse

Source: From the Illustrated London News of November 22, 1919.

no trouble finding confirming empirical evidence. He points to Marxist theory of history, Freudian psychoanalysis, and Adler's individual psychology as prime examples of pseudo-sciences that apparently enjoyed a great deal of empirical confirmation. Soothsayers, like astrologers, can make their predictions so utterly vague that no matter how the future unfolds, their predictions will come true.

Marxist theorists of history, Popper argues, behave similarly. They find evidence to confirm their theories of class struggle everywhere they look, from newspapers to religion. Worse yet:

> in spite of the serious efforts of some of its founders and followers, [the theory] ultimately adopted this soothsaying practice. In some of its earlier formulations (for example in Marx's analysis of the character of the 'coming social revolution') their predictions were testable and, in fact, falsified. Yet instead of accepting the refutations, the followers of Marx re-interpreted both the theory and the evidence in order to make them agree.
>
> *(Popper, 2002, p. 49)*

By revising predictions so that they always match with empirical observations, Popper argues, Marxist theorists give up the scientific status of the Marxist theory of history for a never-ending stream of empirical confirmations.

Freudian psychoanalysis and Adler's individual psychology suffer from similar defects. By continually making post-hoc revisions, Popper argues that these theories could interpret any empirical observations as being consistent with the theories. Contrary to the opinions of their proponents, this immunity from falsity, Popper claims, constitutes their gravest weakness.[6]

Contrast these theories with the progress made by early 20th century physics. Einstein, for instance, famously claimed in 1916 that the paths of light can be affected by gravitational attraction. If his theory was correct, one should be able to observe light "bending" around massive objects. Fortunately, a solar eclipse was set to occur in 1919, which allowed for the observation of the effects of starlight as it traveled past the darkened and massive sun, thus giving Einstein a perfect opportunity to test his theory. The British scientist Arthur Eddington led an expedition to the tiny island of Principe off the coast of West Africa (in addition to sending another team to Brazil) to observe the eclipse and to determine if Einstein's predictions were correct. The stunning results became the first set of empirical evidence confirming Einstein's general theory of relativity.

Unlike the Marxist theory of history, psychoanalysis, and individual psychology, the predictions entailed by general relativity were concrete and "risky." Eddington could have made observations that were clearly inconsistent with Einstein's predictions. Popper argues that it is this aspect of Einstein's general relativity that makes it a genuine science. What distinguishes science from pseudo-science is precisely that the former contains claims that are falsifiable.

TABLE 1.2 Popper's logic of falsification

1)	H → O
2)	~O
	~H

H = hypothesis
O = observation

While confirmation relies on inductive inference, falsification is deductive; that is, if an observation is inconsistent with a prediction, we can conclude definitively (and not merely probably) that the theory that produces the prediction is false. By relying on falsifiability as the difference between science and pseudo-science, Popper hopes to avoid the objections that he raises against inductive logic as the logic of science.

The legacy of Popper's falsifiability criterion continues to hold sway in much of the contemporary understanding of science and medicine. In advocating for the need for supporting empirical evidence to validate a psychotherapy, cognitive scientist Daniel David and behavioral oncologist Guy Montgomery, for instance, suggest that "validating a theory refers to testing it, based on a current scientific approach (e.g., falsifiability, verifiability)" (David & Montgomery, 2011, p. 92). Likewise, Italian psychologists Barbara Treccani and Claudio Mulatti argue that the absence of a clear understanding of the cognitive mechanism guiding bilingualism prevents one from making "precise, univocal and *falsifiable* predictions about the possible effects of bilingualism on cognition, brain structure and cerebral functioning," and this fact partially explains why "this line of research has great difficulties in moving away from the unstructured, chaotic stage that necessarily characterizes the initial investigations of a given phenomenon to enter into a more mature phase" (Treccani & Mulatti, 2015, p. 351. My emphasis.). Oxford physicist David Grimes similarly extolls the epistemic virtue of falsifiability in his discussion of the public acceptance of conspiracy theories. He writes,

> Conspiratorial ideation is the tendency of individuals to believe that events and power relations are secretly manipulated by certain clandestine groups and organizations. Many of these ostensibly explanatory conjectures are non-falsifiable, lacking in evidence or demonstrably false, yet public acceptance remains high.
>
> *(Grimes, 2016, p. 1)*

The biostatistician Stephen Senn relies on Popper's falsificationism to argue that "[t]he clinical trial is designed with refutation in mind; its ability to corroborate is of necessity more limited since blinding, randomization and control only reveal their value fully in the case of refutation" (Senn, 1991, p. 1691). In other words, the aim of clinical trials is to attempt to falsify a hypothesis—exactly as Popper suggests.

It is important to keep in mind that using falsifiability to distinguish science from pseudo-science is not just a philosophical exercise. Millions of research dollars are at stake, in addition to decisions by insurance companies and federal agencies to cover alternative and complementary medical treatments.[7] The issue goes farther than whether alternative and complementary treatments are effective. Just because something improves a person's health, it does not follow that it falls within the domain of *scientific* medicine. For example, although there is robust evidence that poverty and health are intimately linked, improving someone's economic status, even with the goal of improving his or her health, does not clearly fall within the traditional purview of medicine. If a practice is not scientific, and if we take modern medicine to be grounded in science, then it follows that said practice is not a part of modern medicine, regardless of its efficacy in improving one's health. Knowing whether something is a science or not, therefore, is a necessary step in determining whether it is a part of modern medicine.

1.5 Holism Ends Falsifiability

Popper's falsifiability criterion, alas, faces a number of serious problems. Like verificationism, falsifiability would rule out any theoretical sciences that do not generate empirical predictions as genuine sciences (e.g., some areas of theoretical physics). A deeper problem, however, is that falsifiability seems to do a poor job of capturing what scientists *actually* do. More specifically, when scientists observe experimental results that differ from their expectations, they do not immediately conclude that the experiments have falsified their theories. Instead, they attempt to identify the assumptions that they made in designing and conducting the experiments and they look to reject these secondary assumptions while preserving the core principles. In other words, rather than testing a hypothesis in isolation, a scientist always tests the hypothesis together with other auxiliary assumptions. Some of these assumptions are theoretical (e.g., the laws of optics that guide the use of a microscope) and some of them are practical (e.g., the lenses of the microscope are clean).

TABLE 1.3 Actual logic of falsification

1)	$(H \,\&\, A_1 \,\&\, A_2 \,\&\, A_3 \ldots A_n) \rightarrow O$
2)	$\sim O$
	$\sim(H \,\&\, A_1 \,\&\, A_2 \,\&\, A_3 \ldots A_n)$

H = hypothesis
O = observation
A_n = auxiliary assumptions

And, we might very well not know all the assumptions we are implicitly making. When the results are not what the experimenters expected, they do not immediately reject their target hypothesis. On the contrary, they reexamine the totality of their assumptions and they call into question the assumption(s) that led to the failed prediction. While Popper believes that scientific hypotheses are and can be tested in isolation such that false predictions deductively entail falsified hypotheses, the reality of science shows that hypotheses are never tested in isolation. Scientific testing is a far more holistic exercise than Popper suggests. When an experiment fails to produce the predicted observation, all we can deduce is that the conglomerate of hypothesis and the host of auxiliary assumptions contain something false. We cannot deduce exactly where the falsity lies.

One of the earliest philosophers of science to notice the impossibility of testing hypotheses in isolation was the French physicist and philosopher of science Pierre Duhem. In his *The Aim and Structure of Physical Theory*, he states:

> In sum, the physicist can never subject an isolated hypothesis to experimental test, but only a whole group of hypotheses; when the experiment is in disagreement with his predictions, what he learns is that at least one of the hypotheses constituting this group is unacceptable and ought to be modified; but the experiment does not designate which one should be changed.
> *(Duhem, 1991, p. 149)*

Duhem must have anticipated an uncomfortable consequence of his holistic view of theory-testing. If he were correct, after all, it would be difficult to see how logic and scientific experiments alone can help us identify the rotten apples that are responsible for the false predictions. His attempt to salvage the rationality of experimentation led him to suggest that there are "motives which do not proceed from logic and yet direct our choices. . . . These 'reasons which reason does not know' . . . constitute what is appropriately called good sense" (Duhem, 1991, p. 217). It is unfortunate that Duhem does not further explain exactly what scientific "good sense" consists of and how one might come to possess and to deploy it properly. As is often the case, Pascal's memorable phrase "reasons which reason does not know" marks a gap in the argument.[8]

Historians of science often cite the discovery of Neptune by Urbain Le Verrier of France and John Adams of England, working independently in 1845, to illustrate the holistic nature of scientific investigation. Since William Hershel's observation of Uranus in the late 18th century, astronomers knew that Uranus' orbit did not behave as Newton's celestial mechanics had predicted. Its irregularities could not be explained by Newton's laws of gravitation. According to Popper's picture of science, Newton's laws entail false predictions and should thus be rejected. Nevertheless, an entire generation of astronomers held on to Newton's laws and looked to explain Uranus' irregularities by exploring other possibilities.

Le Verrier and Adams noticed that most astronomers at the time believed that Uranus was the last planet in our solar system. Nevertheless, if this assumption was incorrect, the gravitational pull of another (unseen) planet farther from the sun than Uranus could explain Uranus' irregularities. Using nothing but the perturbation of Uranus' orbit, Le Verrier and Adams calculated the mass and orbit of a hypothetical (and unseen) planet. The proposed planet was observed and their predictions confirmed a year later in 1846, and it was later named Neptune (proposed by Le Verrier, whose eponymous suggestion to name the planet "Le Verrier" was rejected earlier).

What this historic episode shows is that scientists do not reject their core beliefs (e.g., Newton's laws) in the face of false predictions. Moreover, hypotheses cannot be tested one at a time. Empirical falsification (and verification) can only be done in a holistic manner in which one's hypotheses are tested together with a host of auxiliary assumptions. In this respect, Popper's idea that falsifiability is the key defining characteristic of scientific claim fails to match up with the holistic nature of empirical testing.[9] Falsifiability cannot be the real difference between science and pseudo-science because falsifiability with its testing of hypotheses in isolation, as Popper has proposed, is in principle impossible to do.

1.6 The Wrath of Kuhn

One of the nice features of Popper's view is that if we have a clear understanding of the principles and methodological structures of a discipline, we can tell if the discipline logically entails any falsifiable predictions; i.e., we can *a priori* (without appealing to any empirical evidence) tell if a discipline is a science. The idea that we can look "internally" and determine a discipline's scientific status is a holdover from the positivists' desire to uncover the logic of science. If to be a science is to investigate the world using some specific system of logic, then we can tell *a priori* if the investigation is scientific. The actual practice of scientists becomes philosophically unimportant.

The publication of Thomas Kuhn's *The Structure of Scientific Revolution* (*SSR*) in 1962, however, fundamentally changed how we study and view the nature of science. While previous philosophers certainly knew much of the history and practice of science, Kuhn's careful examination of some of the most iconic scientific breakthroughs shows that the practice and the progression of science are not guided by any clean logic of discovery. Kuhn instead argues that extra-scientific factors such as political forces, institutional resources, the presence of charismatic proponents, and so on often dictate the direction of scientific revolution. In order for us to better appreciation Kuhn's view, it is important that we understand Kuhn's idea of the different stages of science development.

According to Kuhn, a scientific discipline does not evolve in a smooth and gradual manner—that is, slowly accumulating new knowledge and discarding false ideas. A science, instead, moves through a series of stages. A discipline begins in a pre-scientific stage in which practitioners do not agree on a shared outlook; that is, they do not agree on the fundamental principles, central research issues, criteria for an adequate solution to a research problem, and so on. From this chaotic stage, a paradigm may emerge to guide the practice of a discipline and usher in the normal science stage. Normal science is characterized by the presence of a paradigm. Kuhn's concept of a paradigm consists of two major components: (1) a scientific outlook, and (2) exemplars that best illustrate what it is to be a good scientist in the discipline. What constitutes an outlook for a science is more than just a set of core theoretical commitments. It also includes extra-scientific elements, such as how professional qualifications are granted, what research problems are legitimate, what metaphysical assumptions are acceptable (e.g., can there be spooky stuff in one's theories?), which recalcitrant problems practitioners can ignore, what constitutes an acceptable result (e.g., peer-reviewed publications), and so on. When a discipline develops a paradigm, it moves from a pre-scientific stage to a normal science stage.

In normal science, practitioners do not attempt to undermine or falsify core theories. On the contrary, day-to-day science is characterized by a conservative and painfully slow approach of solving small puzzles that seem to conflict with the paradigm. It is this puzzle-solving tradition within the confines of a paradigm that marks the presence of a normal science, Kuhn argues. In this sense, *any* discipline can be a science as long as there exists a paradigm that allows for a puzzle-solving tradition. What distinguishes a science from a pseudo-science lies not with any internal theoretical structure of the discipline—a logic of science, *pace* Popper and the positivists. It lies, instead, with the presence of certain real-world features (like clear definition of what constitutes professional qualifications) that help define a paradigm. It turns out, science is as science does.

A normal science, however, does not necessarily endure forever. At some point, recalcitrant problems might become significant enough that they bring along a crisis in the science. A new approach might emerge promising to solve the crisis and return the discipline to a normal stage. Kuhn controversially argues that the selection of a new paradigm is not based on any rational logic. Scientific revolutions are akin to religious conversions and political revolutions. Regime changes, even when driven by grassroot efforts, might not lead to a "better" political system. The very idea that there is a recipe to a successful result is implausible at best. Scientific revolutions, like all grand social changes, are messy and unpredictable.

The publication of *SSR* has radically changed how we understand and study the nature of science. Kuhn's work has certainly spelled the end for verificationism and falsificationism. The idea that a discipline is clearly not scientific because it does not offer falsifiable observations is no longer taken to be true. Furthermore, Kuhn also casts serious doubts as to whether there is such a thing as the logic of scientific discovery (independent of sociopolitical factors). The days of being able to examine the inner theoretical structure of a discipline and determine *a priori* its scientific status are most definitely over.

1.7 Science: What Is It Good For?

We began our chapter with a discussion of the scientific status of medicine. And we conclude that empirical verification or falsifiability cannot be sufficient (and perhaps not even necessary) for something to be considered a science. We have assumed up to now that medicine ought to be scientific. One of Kuhn's legacies is that there is no sharp theoretical line between science and non-science; any practice—from material physics to witchcraft—with a sufficiently robust paradigm can be a science. If he is correct, then grounding medicine in science becomes less epistemically special.

To be sure, Kuhn is an admirer and proponent of science, but his respect stems from the practical results that science delivers. He prefers modern science to, say, witchcraft not because there is something fundamentally superior about the former; rather, science is better because it gives us the things that we want (e.g., higher quality of life, more happiness, longevity, etc.). From the point of view of medical care, if a particular therapy improves our well-being, whether it is rooted in modern science is secondary. A medicine grounded in this Kuhnian view of science would place pragmatic outcomes above the scientific status of a practice.[10]

Our trust in modern medicine is partly based on the belief that it differs from other modes of healing because science is epistemically special. If it turns out, as Kuhn argues, that science is special only from a pragmatic point of view, then the rejections or dismissals of treatments considered "non-scientific" are premature. A treatment that "works" would be consistent with the spirit of a pragmatic justification of science and it would also encourage us to rethink our paradigm to ensure that normal science can incorporate non-traditional modalities: it would make for a smart move for those who wish to defend the superiority of science on pragmatic grounds.

Most importantly, we need to reflect on what we mean by "works." There is no doubt that modern medicine and public health at large have accomplished some remarkable things. The Oxford Martin Programme on Global Development at the University of Oxford (Roser, 2018) estimates that the global child mortality rate (death before the age of 5) has plummeted from 43.3% in 1800 to 4.25% in 2015. Millions and millions of children are spared from early deaths and needless suffering because of medicine and public health efforts. At the same time, if we want to provide a pragmatic justification for medicine and science, we need to identify first what they are supposed to deliver, and then determine whether they in fact do a good job delivering them. The first question is really a not-so-subtly disguised question about what we want in life. Are we better off now than we were a hundred years ago? Do we live more meaningful and enriching lives with a greater ability and more time to do what we want to do? I will let readers consider their answers to these fundamental questions about our existence.

We will return to the more manageable epistemic questions such as "How do we know if a treatment works?" and "What justifies our reliance on evidence?"

in subsequent chapters. Before then, let's look at the fascinating question of what makes a human condition a disease as opposed to a mere variation in our species. Like the scientific status of modern medicine, the definition of disease and health will be of deep philosophical interest and will affect the practice of medicine both clinically and research-wise.

Notes

1 If the idea of a physician recommending higher education for mental health purposes seems far-fetched, consider the now typical practice of a physician asking if her patients wear seatbelts or bicycle helmets.

2 The Spanish Influenza must have affected many of the leading positivists personally. The philosopher Ludwig Wittgenstein, whose work radically shaped Anglo-American analytic philosophy in the 20th century, grew up in a privileged and notable home in Vienna. A servant of his family died from the flu. The Viennese artist Egon Schiele—a gifted student of Gustav Klimt, and a contemporary of Wittgenstein—fell by the flu at the age of 28, three days after his wife Edith, who was carrying their child, also died from the flu. Klimt was a patron of the Wittgenstein family, and he painted a portrait for Ludwig's older sister Margaret Stonborough-Wittgenstein for her wedding. Little has been written on the impact of the Spanish Influenza on the intellectual development of positivism. One suspects that the terrifying efficiency by which the flu killed must have prompted many to look to modern science for salvation.

3 A religious statement, such as "God exists," would have no meaning if there were no empirical consequences that one could derive from it. Likewise, some positivists argued that moral statements like "Murder is wrong" also have no empirical consequences. According to the verificationist theory of meaning, these sentences are not just not true—they are literally meaningless.

4 Pseudo-sciences are not necessarily spooky, either. There might be purely physicalistic explanations for claims made in phrenology. These explanations do not require supernatural phenomena or interactions. What makes phrenology a pseudo-science—indeed, what makes *anything* a pseudo-science—is not that the discipline contains the supernatural, per se.

5 This is, of course, a simplification. Correlations do not necessarily reveal causal connections. We also need to look at how the proposed causal connection coheres with our other accepted beliefs about the working of the world. A full discussion of the nature of causation will come later, but it is worth noting that to understand the world in terms of causal connections *requires* that we begin with some observed correlations. Causations are not things that we can observe directly; they are things that we infer. Causations are, in this sense, built up from correlations.

6 A number of scholars have called into question Popper's characterization of these theories. For a fascinating discussion on Popper and psychoanalysis, especially how Freud revised his view in light of new evidence (*pace* Popper's claim), see (Grant & Harari, 2005).

7 In a March 17th 2009 piece in the *Washington Post* titled "Scientists Speak Out Against Federal Funds for Research on Alternative Medicine," the author David Brown states that the National Institute of Health has an annual research budget of $300 million earmarked for research in alternative and complementary treatments.

8 The line first made its appearance in Pascal's *Pensées*, published posthumously in 1670. The original French, "Le cœur a ses raisons, que la raison ne connaît point," can be roughly translated as "The heart has its reasons, which reason does not know."

9 Although the formal logic of empirical falsification as Popper envisioned turned out to be incorrect, one can see the spirit behind Popper's proposal. Intuitively, science prides

itself on being open-minded; that is, it allows for the possibility that even the most cherished dogma is false. Pseudo-science (especially theories that aim to insulate themselves from ever being false) seems to embrace dogmatism and allegiance come-what-may. Perhaps it is science's apparent anti-dogmatism that Popper noticed, and offered falsifiability (albeit, incorrectly) as a way to capture the sentiment. Alas, the belief that modern science is open-minded is also questionable in light of some of Thomas Kuhn's views.

10 To be sure, whether modern science has actually made our lives better is a difficult question to answer. As much as we live longer and healthier lives, modern science has also introduced weapons of mass destruction that place the lives of more people at existential risk than at any other time in the history of humanity. If the special status of science is measured by its pragmatic usefulness, then it is an empirical question whether it is in fact special.

References

David, D., & Montgomery, G. H. (2011). The scientific status of psychotherapies: A new evaluative framework for evidence-based psychosocial interventions. *Clinical Psychology: Science and Practice, 18*(2), 89–99. doi:10.1111/j.1468-2850.2011.01239.x

Duhem, P. M. M., Wiener, P. P., Vuillemin, J., & de Broglie, L. (1991). *The aim and structure of physical theory*. Princeton, NJ: Princeton University Press.

Glymour, C., & Stalker, D. (1983). Engineers, cranks, physicians, magicians. *New England Journal of Medicine, 308*(16), 960–964. doi:10.1056/NEJM198304213081611

Grant, D. C., & Harari, E. (2005). Psychoanalysis, science and the seductive theory of Karl Popper. *Australian and New Zealand Journal of Psychiatry, 39*(6), 446–452. doi:10.1080/j.1440-1614.2005.01602.x

Grimes, D. R. (2016). On the viability of conspiratorial beliefs. *PLoS ONE, 11*(1), e0147905. doi:10.1371/journal.pone.0147905

Mach, E. (1988). *The science of mechanics: A critical and historical account of its development* (T. McCormack, Trans.). Open Court.

Popper, K. R. (2002). *Conjectures and refutations: The growth of scientific knowledge*. London and New York, NY: Routledge.

Roser, M. (2018). *Child mortality*. Retrieved from https://ourworldindata.org/child-mortality

Senn, S. (1991). Falsification and clinical trials. *Statistics in Medicine, 10*, 1679–1692.

Sicher, F., Targ, E., Moore, D., & Smith, H. S. (1998). A randomized double-blind study of the effect of distant healing in a population with advanced AIDS: Report of a small scale study. *Western Journal of Medicine, 169*(6), 356–363.

Treccani, B., & Mulatti, C. (2015). No matter who, no matter how . . . and no matter whether the white matter matters: Why theories of bilingual advantage in executive functioning are so difficult to falsify. *Cortex, 73*, 349–351. doi:http://dx.doi.org/10.1016/j.cortex.2015.07.015

Walsemann, K. M., Bell, B. A., & Hummer, R. A. (2012). Effects of timing and level of degree attained on depressive symptoms and self-rated health at midlife. *American Journal of Public Health, 102*(3), 557–563. doi:10.2105/AJPH.2011.300216

2

THE CONCEPT OF HEALTH

2.1 Are You Sick or Are You Just Different?

There clearly exists a close connection between the practice of medicine and the concept of health. Both research medicine and clinical care aim to improve our health. But what exactly constitutes health and, relatedly, diseases and disabilities? There are biological variations that we do not believe fall into the domain of diseases. For instance, having curly hair is a biological (specifically, genetic) trait; yet, no one would think of it as a disease. Hemophilia—a condition that leads to potentially fatal delays in blood clotting—is a hereditary disease caused by mutations in the patients' genes. It would be odd to say that human beings, like the curliness of one's hair, come into two natural varieties: hemophiliac and non-hemophiliac. The definition of health is thus really a question about what constitutes natural variants within our species.

From a practical point of view, the definition of health affects questions such as whether a condition warrants medical treatment, whether one is morally responsible for the behaviors caused by it, and whether the state and insurance providers are required to pay for treatment. In 2011, activists and researchers held a symposium at Syracuse University to advocate for a change in how we understand autism. Rather than seeing it as a disease, advocates suggested that we ought to think of autism as a different but natural form of human cognition. The National Symposium on Neurodiversity issued the following statement:

> Neurodiversity is a concept where neurological differences are to be recognized and respected as any other human variation. These differences can include those labeled with Dyspraxia, Dyslexia, Attention Deficit Hyperactivity Disorder, Dyscalculia, Autistic Spectrum, Tourette Syndrome, and others.
>
> For many autistic people, neurodiversity is viewed is a concept and social movement that advocates for viewing autism as a variation of human

TABLE 2.1 A truncated family tree of Queen Victoria showing the hemophiliac path

By the eve of World War I, the monarchs of three major participating countries (Germany, England, and Russia) were cousins—all descendants of Queen Victoria. The proliferation of Victoria's family line in Europe also meant that many of her descendants inherited her hemophiliac gene. From Prince Waldemar of Prussia to Alfonso—Prince of Asturias the heir-apparent of Spain—the deaths of Queen Victoria's descendants (caused by uncontrollable bleeding) virtually wiped out the major royal lines in Europe. The old practice of cementing political power by marrying across royal houses might have ironically spelled their doom.

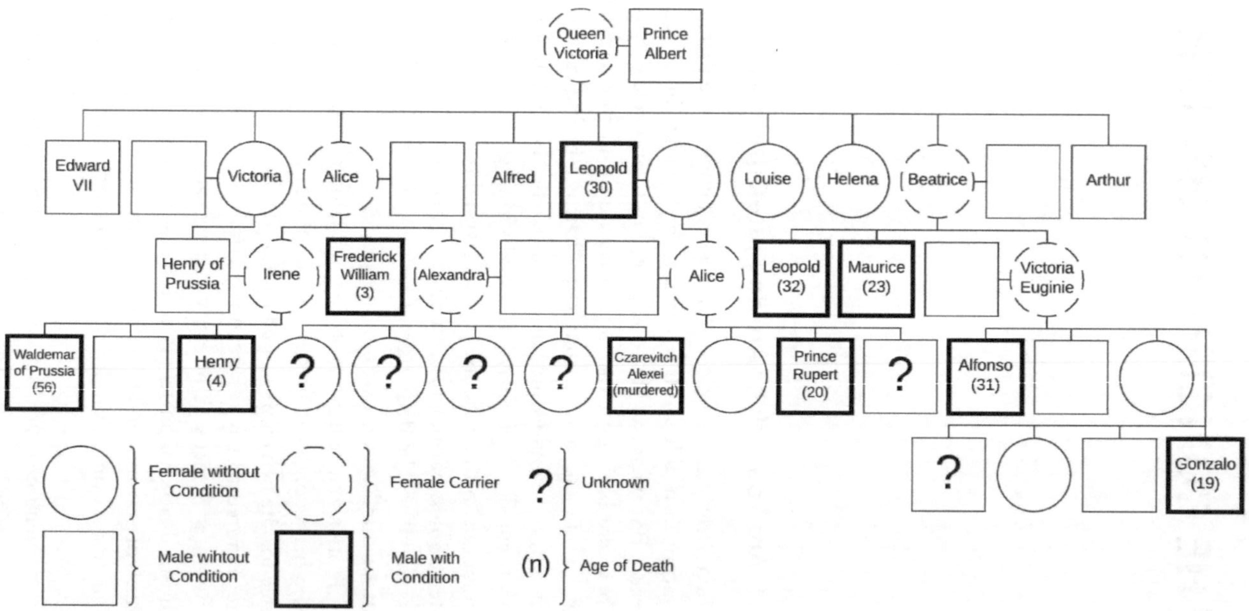

> wiring, rather than a disease. As such, neurodiversity activists reject the idea that autism should be cured, advocating instead for celebrating autistic forms of communication and self-expression, and for promoting support systems that allow autistic people to live as autistic people.
>
> *(2011)*

Viewing autism as a "natural" evolution of the human species, proponents of autism-*qua*-neurodiversity eschew spending resources to identify the causes of and the cure for the condition. Being autistic is akin to being tall, having detached earlobes, or having darker skin color; albeit, autists have many more challenges in a society with neurotypical norms. Advocates of autist rights, however, argue that these difficulties come from implicit and explicit neurotypical biases. Just as the Civil Rights Movement recognized and fought for the rights of racial minorities, we too should recognize and fight for the rights of neuro-minorities.[1]

The pivoting that we see in autism is but one of many examples of how we continually rethink what constitutes a healthy human being. After more than a decade of debate, the American Psychiatric Association finally removed homosexuality from the Diagnostic and Statistical Manual of Mental Disorders in 1987; the World Health Organization followed suit in 1993. (We will return to this topic later.) Recently, a fertility clinic in New England was asked by a couple to help them create an embryo with Down syndrome. Neither of the parents-to-be had Down syndrome; they simply wanted a Down positive child. Their argument centered around the belief that Down syndrome should not be thought of as a disease but as a normal neurological variant. If the selection of genotypical traits like sex falls under the umbrella of reproductive autonomy, so the argument goes, then surely these parents-to-be have the right to choose to have a child with Down.

The question of what constitutes health and what constitutes "non-health" (a broad term that includes illnesses, diseases, and disabilities) affects a wide gamut of social practices from medicine to political rights. The Americans with Disabilities Act (ADA) of 1990, for instance, not only prohibits discrimination against individuals with disabilities, it also mandates reasonable accommodations by both private and public organizations to ensure that these individuals have equal access to services. By ensuring adequate accommodations, ADA attempts to restore parity; that is, ADA aims to eliminate the disparity in opportunities between the disabled individuals and non-disabled by providing the necessary supports for the former.[2] The underlying assumption is that social and political opportunities that we are entitled to are set by the range a healthy individual is capable of pursuing. The philosophical reason for this is obvious: we are physical beings and our autonomy and liberty are limited by our typical healthy physiology (Cartesian disembodied spirits notwithstanding!). If we are to know what a typical person is capable of doing, we need to establish what constitutes a healthy person. In this respect, the question of health really touches on some of the deepest philosophical questions about what we fundamentally are.

In the current philosophy of medicine literature, there are two broad approaches to defining health: health is either a value-free or a value-laden concept. For the first approach, one might define health on the basis of some objective, biological, or statistical facts about us. For instance, one might say that a person is healthy if and only if her physiology is functioning in a manner typical of our species. The basic idea of this approach is that we can define the concept of health using only scientific concepts and descriptions. According to proponents of this approach, health is a purely biological notion.[3]

For the second approach, the definition of health necessarily includes references to values. We can think of values as the worth or desirability of something; typical examples include happiness, autonomy, meaningful interpersonal relationships, money, or knowledge. Some of these things might be valuable in and of themselves (intrinsically valuable), while others are valuable because they can deliver things that are valuable (instrumentally valuable). Money, for instance, is instrumentally valuable because of its ability to acquire happiness. The moment money ceases to be able to do this (say, during a zombie outbreak), it loses its value. A value-laden definition of health might define health in terms of the physiological conditions necessary to deliver something we consider valuable (e.g., happiness). To be healthy is to be able to acquire and maintain things that are valuable. One attractive feature of this approach is that it can easily explain why we care about being healthy: health is valuable because of its ability to secure other valuable things like longevity and autonomy. In other words, health is of great instrumental value.

2.2 Two Basic Ways to Define Health and Disease

On one end of the spectrum, philosophers such as Christopher Boorse, Paul Thagard, and Norman Daniels attempt to provide value-free analyses of health and disease in terms of biological or empirical facts alone. Boorse (1997) defines a disease as a statistically species-subnormal biological part-function. For instance, a middle-aged man is healthy if and only if his biological parts are functioning efficiently on typical occasions to produce statistically normal results that contribute to his survival and reproduction. If his pancreas, for instance, fails to produce a statistically normal amount of insulin relative to men of his age such that it threatens his survival or reproduction, then he is diseased. In a similar vein, Daniels suggests that "disease and disability . . . are construed as adverse departures from or impairments of species-typical normal functional organization" (2000, p. 314).

Both of these definitions of health rely on bald biological facts with minimal or no reference to values. This approach is often referred to as naturalism or objectivism. The basic motivation behind it is that health and disease are facts about the internal biological functioning of our bodies. When the internal functioning deviates from the normal range, we are ill. This might be so even if the deviation does not affect our behavior, range of social opportunity, or subjective sense of well-being.

Coming from the opposite end of the spectrum, theorists like Rachel Cooper, Tristram Engelhardt, Lawrie Reznek, and Caroline Whitbeck argue that health and disease can be understood only in terms of our values. These value-laden views are sometime referred to as normativism or constructivism. For example, Cooper (2002) argues that a disease must satisfy three conditions:

(1) The condition must be a bad thing for the sufferer;
(2) The sufferer must be unlucky; and
(3) The condition must be potentially medically treatable.

Take a person who has inherited one gene for sickle cell anemia. She has sickle cell trait (SCT) but does not have any of the symptoms of sickle cell anemia. Although she can pass on the sickle cell recessive gene to her children, her SCT provides some level of immunity against malaria (something that she values). According to Cooper, SCT would not be a disease for this particular woman (by condition (1). Of course, if it turns out that she values not passing the gene to her children over increased immunity to malaria, then it would be a different matter.

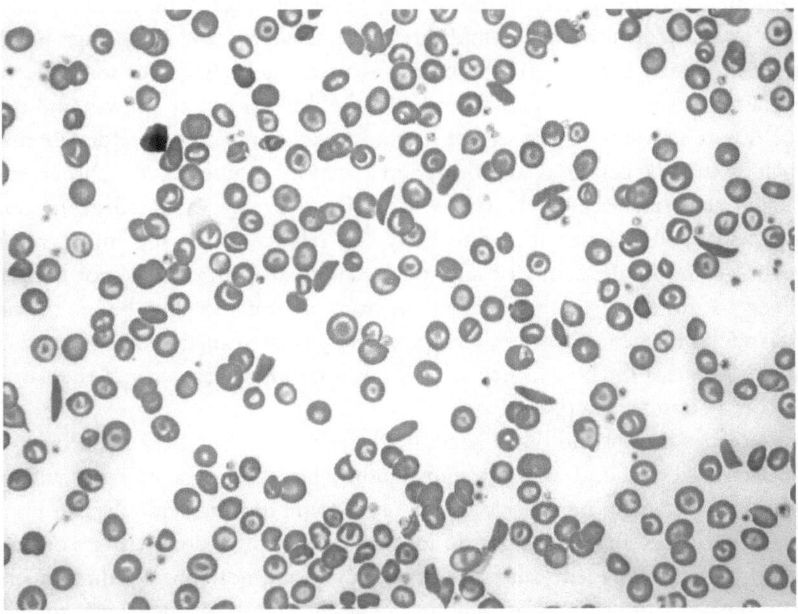

FIGURE 2.1 Sickle Cells

While normal red blood cells are round, individuals with sickle cell anemia have blood cells that resemble sickles (notice the sliver-shaped cells). *Source:* Keith Chambers, Scooter Projet, [CC BY-SA 3.0 (https://creativecommons.org/licenses/by-sa/3.0)], via Wikimedia Commons.

Teething, a painful phase for children, is also not a disease because we would not consider someone unlucky to be teething. In fact, we might consider not-teething to be an unlucky condition! Finally, being born to poor parents might be bad for the person's health outcomes, and we might even consider it a stroke of bad luck. But we do not generally think of poverty as a disease. The reason, Cooper argues, is that poverty is not a medically treatable condition, and thus fails the third condition.

Cooper's analysis represents a prime example of a normativist definition of health. The defining characteristic of normativism is that some social or personal value must play an indispensable role in explicating health and disease. What makes a particular physiological condition a disease accordingly is that the condition must negatively impact the patient's ability to acquire things that are valuable. In other words, there is no objective biological way to determine if a given physiological condition is a disease. All diseases are diseases only relative to a set of values of the patient or the community. The same physiological condition might be a disease in one context and a non-disease in another. The difference lies in how the condition affects the person's values. In a literate society, for instance, dyslexia might be a disorder because we value literacy. The same condition in a non-literate community obviously wouldn't even surface and therefore would not be considered a disease.

Another way to appreciate the difference between naturalism and normativism is to consider how they would categorize asymptomatic early-stage prostate cancer in elderly patients. By definition, prostate cancer involves some form of neoplasm; that is, there is a deviation from the normal rate of growth and death of cells leading to the emergence of tumors. A naturalist account of disease might conclude that the patient is suffering from a disease because his condition consists of some abnormal cellular behaviors (as defined by the intended evolutionary purposes of cells) or that it is statistically rare relative to the sex and age of the patient.[4] To be sure, a naturalist might concede that treatments are not necessary perhaps because the patient will likely die from other pathologies before the neoplasm affects him. Nevertheless, asymptomatic prostate cancer, however dormant, still indicates that the body is not behaving as it should and, as a result, the naturalists would consider it a disease.

A normativist, on the other hand, might conclude that there is no disease at all because the tissue growth (though unusual) places no limitation on what the patient would otherwise be able to do—it is asymptomatic, after all. The human body experiences lots of changes. So long as these changes do not affect or pose a threat to what the patient values, a normativist would not consider them diseases. Being born with fingers whose lengths fall within the 99.8th percentile might be unusual but not pathological. However, being born with extra fingers (polydactyly) is considered a deformity that may warrant surgical intervention. The rarity of these two conditions is roughly the same (polydactyly affects about 1 in 500 children). We might even imagine that there exists a common underlying biological cause for both conditions (e.g., the presence of certain toxins during pregnancy). Nevertheless, a normativist would conclude that having unusually long fingers is not a disease or a disability while being polydactyl is. The difference ultimately lies in our values such as aesthetics, availability of social opportunities, and personal preferences.

There are of course numerous attempts to blend these two views together to create a hybrid view. One might, for instance, suggest that some diseases like organ failure can be understood in purely biological terms and that some diseases like mental illness must be defined in terms of their impact on our values. Alternatively, one might offer a hybrid view that incorporates both empirical biological facts and values together in defining a specific health and disease. It might say that X is a disease if and only if X has certain empirical characteristics (e.g., statistically rare) *and* X affects some values. As with any hybrid view, there are two general problems. First, if some diseases can be defined as biological and some cannot, we want to know why the distinction exists—why can a purely biological analysis of one not be applied to the other? Secondly, the sort of "internal" hybrid view where one mixes biological facts with values must confront cases when the two conditions conflict. What do we say when a condition is statistically common but significantly affects our values? Consider the concept of a universal disease, that is, a disease that affects everyone. The deterioration of mental acuity as we age is a case in point. It satisfies only one of the two conditions. Thus, it should not be considered a disease. Yet, if we think a condition's impact on our values is an important part of what makes it a disease, it is certainly puzzling and contrary to the spirit of the definition to consider a physiological condition that robs us of valuable things not a disease.

2.3 Some Difficulties of Both Approaches

In order to determine which approach is correct, we want to test it against our commonsensical judgments about diseases and health. After all, if a proposed definition fails to capture the bulk of our judgments about diseases and health, we might rightly be skeptical of it.[5] One central difficulty with a normative theory is that it seems to do a rather poor job of capturing our intuitions about which condition is a disease and which is not. Suppose a normativist offers the simple analysis that X is a disease if and only if we have a negative attitude towards the symptoms of X. Being bald, for instance, would be a disease in a community where baldness is a negative.

The problem here is that there have been plenty of conditions that we used to see as social liabilities that we have come to realize were clearly not diseases at all. For instance, up until the early 20th century, Western nations commonly held the view that healthy women experience no sexual pleasure during intercourse and that they do not have sex drives. Female hysteria became a vague disease term to diagnose what we would today consider sexual frustration. For a woman to have a sex drive was considered abnormal. Manual stimulations performed by doctors and

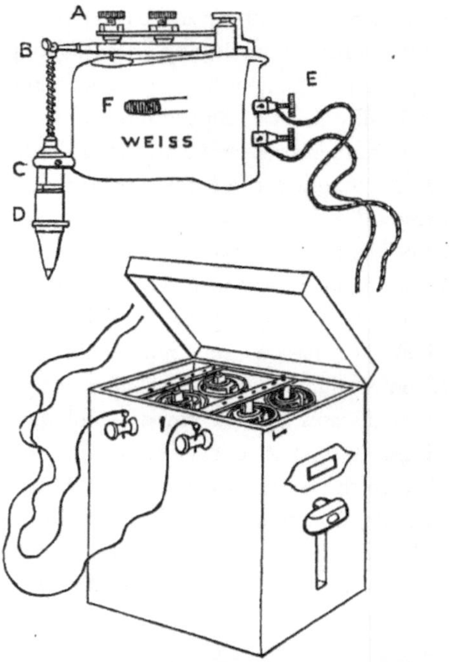

The Percuteur worked by electro-magnetism, and the *Bunsen's Battery*, as supplied by Messrs. Weiss & Sons.

(I am indebted to the late Mr. Donald Napier and Dr. George W. Balfour, of Edinburgh, for the suggestion to use electricity as a motive power for the percuteur.)

E, screws connecting battery wires with the percuteur. A, screws for making connection. There are two; either may be used. That neares the hinge of the vibrator causes the hammer to beat at the highest speed. B, screw for attaching the hammer, brushes, &c., to the instrument. C, brass cylinder through which the rod of the hammer passes. D, vulcanite tube, which is attached with a screw, and regulates the length of the stroke made by the hammer. F, button which, being pressed or pushed with the finger, sets the percuteur going.

FIGURE 2.2 Percuteur

Dr. Mortimer Granville is widely credited for inventing the first battery-operated vibrator (albeit, the battery weighed 40lbs). Nevertheless, he avoided treating female patients for hysteria with it on the grounds that he did not want to be "hoodwinked" by female patients pretending to suffer from the disease (1883, p. 57).

midwives to relieve the symptoms of hysteria led to paroxysms—sudden violent attacks of symptoms including spasms—and not orgasms because many physicians of the time considered the latter biologically impossible for women to experience. A late 19th century woman might see her apparent sex drive as undesirable, abnormal, and socially unacceptable. She might even internalize these values and seek "treatments" to rid herself of them. Yet, we do not want to say that she was sick in any way. As a matter of fact, we feel strongly that she was a healthy woman and that medical professionals, blinded by their cultural sexism, made incorrect diagnoses by medicalizing Victorian values. For normativism, one of the most serious problems is that, for at least some physiological conditions, whether they are diseases or not seems obvious regardless of their effects on social and personal values.

Just as the importance of physiological and biological factors in defining health challenge normativism, the ubiquitous presence of values in medicine poses a similar problem for naturalism as well. Consider homosexuality again. The APA's removal of homosexuality from its list of pathologies in the second edition of its Diagnostic and Statistical Manual (DSM) is considered a moment of great progress in mental health diagnosis. The move was hailed by proponents as long overdue recognition that pathologizing homosexuality justified discrimination and violence against gay people.

Imagine for a moment that researchers discover a common genetic hormonal trait among those who are homosexual. Perhaps the pituitary gland secretes an unusually high amount of hormones, and researchers identify a clear causal pathway that leads most of those who have this trait to be attracted to members of their own gender.[6] If statistical outliers or dysfunctions by an organ (such as subnormal production of hormone) are indicators of a disorder according to naturalism, then homosexuality would be a prima facie pathology. Yet, regardless of how far the functions of the pituitary gland deviate from the norm, we are inclined not to conclude that homosexuality is a disease. The reason for it has less to do with biology than with our values.

Suppose that high intelligence turns out to have a similar underlying causal pathway as homosexuality. Our reluctance to categorize high intelligence as a disease tells us that, for some human conditions, whether they are diseases or not rests *entirely* on our value-attitude towards the "symptoms" of the condition and not on any underlying biological facts. Homosexuality is not a disease because we value the tolerance of diversity in sexual orientation. We see it as a normal variant of our species (much like we see being smart as a normal variant), physiological, evolutionary, or biological "facts" be damned.

Another difficulty for naturalists is the possibility of "universal diseases," which we briefly alluded to in our discussion of hybrid definitions. An environmental toxin, for instance, that affects all members of a species might render a certain physiological impairment statistically normal, but we might not want to conclude that it is not pathological. Tawakol et al. (2017) have recently identified a possible connection between stress and elevated risks of heart attacks. The amygdala reacts to infections and injuries by instructing bone marrow to produce more white blood cells. The stress of modern life, however, can stimulate the amygdala and cause heightened amounts of white blood cells. These cells then form plaques in the arteries, which elevate the person's risks for cardiovascular disease. Our immune response to stress is the result of perfectly functioning bone marrow. From the point of view of physiology, no part of our body is failing to do its job properly. Yet the proper functioning of our bodily system is rendering us unhealthy by raising our risk of heart attacks. To insist that our immune system is healthy even as it is killing us is dogmatic-unto-ludicrous ("Dear patient, you are perfectly healthy and that is why you are suffering and dying"). Indeed, if we can develop a drug that would lessen our immune response to modern stress, we might see it as a great tool for dealing with a public health threat and not an elective enhancement on a par with cosmetic surgery.

Likewise, almost everyone experiences deterioration in eyesight, cognitive abilities, and bone health with age. Diseases of aging present a tricky challenge to naturalists because not only are they statistically common, they can even be evolutionarily selected. From the point of view of classic Darwinism, selection pressure encourages the proliferation of genetic mutations that are conducive to the replication of those genes. Suppose a mutation "front-loads" our body's resources to benefit the health of our earlier selves at the expense of our older selves. If we live in an environment in which most of us would have died before reaching old age, such a front-loading mutation would contain no evolutionary cost: we would be long dead before the front-loading affects our health (and, more importantly, our reproductive ability). Front-loading has been offered as a potential explanation for senescence.[7] Dementia, for instance, might very well be a result of stiffening arteries that are caused by mutations that front-load the availability of calcium favored by natural selection. Age-related dementia is "natural" because it results from genes that maximize our reproductive odds in a world where most of us die young. When the environment changes (e.g., the elimination of certain pathogens or the extension of life-expectancy), these mutations will no longer confer the same degree of evolutionary benefits on our genes. Given enough time, natural selection will likely and eventually lead to other mutations that bestow benefits that affect our health differently (e.g., less front-loading in a world where the average person lives a far longer life). However, until nature catches up with the environmental changes, the mismatch between mutations and health is akin to riding a bicycle in a river: the inefficiency is a state that resulted from operating a system that was never designed for the particular environment. To call this inefficiency the way things normally or naturally are (that is, healthy) is to place a premium on a mismatch between our physiology and our environment. One might rightly wonder why a specific inefficiency per se is worth maintaining or why *any* inefficiency should be worth maintaining in and of itself.

There is a deeper problem with any account of health that defines health on the basis of natural selection. To speak metaphorically, our genes are "interested" in one thing: *their* ability to reproduce. A gene that grants its host an increased ability to reproduce will, by a matter of logic, lead to a greater number of the gene in the next generation (all else being equal). We want to live long and healthy lives. However, if a mutation results in shorter lives but grants the genes a far greater reproductive rate, selection pressure would lead to the presence of more of the mutant genes for each subsequent generation until it establishes a new equilibrium. A concept of health that appeals to evolutionary consideration will always have to confront the reality that the Darwinian interests of our genes are not always the same as our interests. To put it broadly, what is evolutionarily healthy for our genes does not always coincide with what is healthy *for us*. We are, after all, more than the sum of our genetic impetus.

The example of a "selfish" DNA can help illustrate the gap between a gene's interests and our interests. Approximately two-thirds of the human genome consists of transposable elements (Graur, 2015, p. 417). These elements mostly reside in the parts of our DNA that have no effect on our physiology. However, these transposable elements, or transposons, can move around, replicate, and slice and dice our genes, inserting themselves in various segments of our DNA. Very rarely, when transposons alter our DNA, can they confer positive effects on the host. Most of the time, the changes are either benign or have negative effects on the host. The origins of many of these transposons date back millions of years, and they are now a majority of our genome. When they are benign, they are free-riders, changing our gametes and passing themselves along. When they are harmful, they are not just selfish genes but nasty genes, risking the health of the host in their evolutionary track. From the point of view of our evolutionary fitness (and even health), most selfish genes seem to be useless. However, from the point of view of the genes' evolutionary fitness, they are doing quite well, for they somehow have managed to ride along in our genome for millions of years.

One fascinating question is how nasty genes could find a stable home in a genome. Wouldn't the deleterious effects of these genes on their hosts be akin to burning down one's house? How could they stick around for so long if they are bad for their host's survival? One possible answer is that whatever negative effects they might have on our reproductive fitness, they make up for them in their superior abilities to pass themselves onto future generations. In other words, the host might have a shorter and more reproductively challenged life, but if the genes can make up for the shorter window with a greater number of offspring, these nasty genes are still ahead of the evolutionary curve. In a study of *Drosophila melanogaster* (or common fruit flies), Struchiner, Kidwell, and Ribeiro (2005) found just such an example. They discovered that a specific transposon (*P* elements) lowers the reproductive fitness of fruit flies by 19%. Like any genetic traits, there is a 50% chance that a given one is present in a specific gamete. Struchiner et al. noticed instead that *P* elements are present in *70%* of the gametes, which means the transposon is able to increase its odds of being passed on. Even though the presence of *P* elements lowers the host's reproductive fitness, the 20% increased odds of their presence in gametes outweighs the cost to the host. As such, it reaches a stable place among the genomes of generations of fruit flies by rendering these flies less reproductive while making sure that it is more likely to be in a gamete. In essence, the transposon behaves much like a permanent parasite: stringing the host along and making it less fit, all the while looking out for its own agenda.[8]

Not only do transposons transmit vertically by embedding themselves in gametes, they also transmit horizontally.[9] Oliveira, Bao, Martins, and Jurka (2012) identified a mariner transposon that traveled from tree shrew genomes to hedgehogs' about 69 to 100 million years ago. Insects likely played the role of the

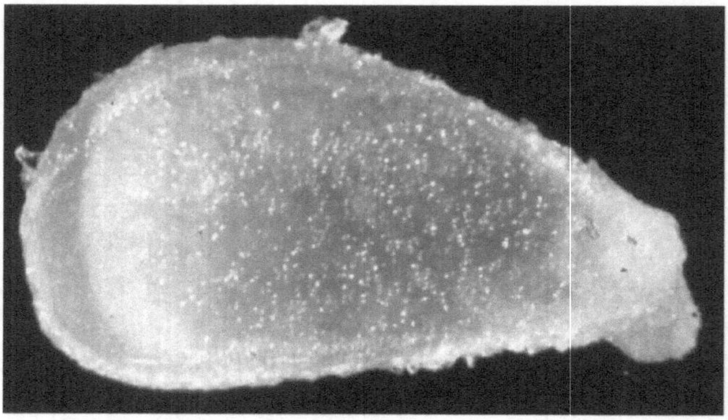

FIGURE 2.3 Cross-section of a Pea Root's Nodule

The darker area in the center (red, in a real sample) indicates the presence of leghemoglobin—another example of horizontal transmission of genetic material. Like its non-plant cousin hemoglobin, leghemoglobin is red in color, structurally similar, and facilitates oxygen storing among the host's cells. Legume plants containing leghemoglobin are able to minimize the level of oxygen so that bacteria around their roots can effectively break down nitrogen into the much-desired ammonia. This ability gives the legume a remarkable advantage. Amazingly, plants do not generally have hemoglobin-type oxygen-transfer proteins. Some researchers have hypothesized that its presence in legumes is the result of horizontal transmission of transposons from bacteria to plants. Manufacturers of meatless burgers have started using leghemoglobin to simulate the "bloodiness" and texture of meat. *Source:* Image from Downie (2005).

intermediary, but the exact mode of transmission remains unclear. By moving horizontally, Oliveira et al. speculate that the mariner transposons managed to avoid reproductive pressure and subsequent extinction. Horizontal transmission of transposons means that, all else being equal, natural selection would favor those genes that are more capable of transmitting across organisms than those that do not. In other words, the constant evolutionary pressure on the transposons would give those that can transmit horizontally an edge over those that cannot. So long as these transposons transmit successfully enough (horizontally), the harm that they do to their host is no threat to their genetic survival. To borrow a popular (albeit, slightly misleading) metaphor, we can think of the host as a bus and the host's genes as the passengers. Nasty transposons that can transmit horizontally are like passengers who have no qualms trashing the bus provided that their hooliganism actually helps them find another bus to hop onto and take them where they want to go.

The fact that transposons make up the bulk of our DNA and have been embedded in us for eons make them no longer temporary residents but a part of our genome. They are like obnoxious manipulative family members whom we can't get rid of. When philosophers speak of the evolutionary purpose of a subsystem or a genotype in our genome, they must include these transposons. Although some of them provide benefits to the host (or more accurately, the parts of our genome that have phenotypical expressions), many of them are either benign or nasty. Their evolutionary purposes do not coincide with ours, let alone our health. The complexity of our genes, filled with fossil genes left over from our ancestors and transposons of all stripes, means that the idea of there being clear and unified evolutionary purposes is unsustainable. It is like looking at Grand Central Station and asking about *the* destination where everyone wishes to go. Worse still, some of the travelers might work against you to ensure that they get to their destinations at your expense. From this chaotic jumble we emerge, and it is important to remember that not everything in our body put there by natural selection has our best interests in mind.

2.4 A Pre-Sliced Nature

One of the philosophical motivations behind the naturalist approach to health and disease is that they are grounded in biology independent of human values or interests. According to this view, the biological world, metaphorically speaking, comes pre-cut at the joints. These objective natural categories are sometimes referred to in philosophy as "natural kinds." In chemistry, we might say that carbon and acid are natural kinds. The intuition is that of all the things that belong to the kind carbon, there is something common among them (e.g., they have a certain atomic number) and this commonality is independent of our values and interests. The concept "sandwich" is not a natural kind, even though there might be some common properties among all sandwiches. The reason is that the concept of a sandwich is dependent on our interests.

With regards to health and disease, a naturalist might be tempted to map health and diseases onto these objective categories in the world. This approach is particularly attractive for those working in research medicine. In studying human physiology, researchers attempt to discover the functions of various parts and subsystems. From red blood cells to the pancreas, research medicine aims to tell us how these things work and, subsequently, how we can manipulate and repair them. To find out how, say, a human liver functions, we need to draw a line separating normal and healthy functions from abnormal and unhealthy ones. The study of physiology, therefore, requires that we have an idea of what constitutes a healthy liver. One obvious way to do this is to pigeonhole biological parts and subsystems along the lines drawn by natural kinds.

Although philosophers disagree on the exact definition of natural kinds, there are some basic ideas that most philosophers would agree to. Natural kinds should:

(1) Group things together that have some shared properties;
(2) Participate in laws of nature; and
(3) Be capable of some inductive projections.

Condition (1) is fairly obvious. Whatever natural kinds are, members of a natural kind should have some common properties. This is of course a necessary but not sufficient condition since *any* two things can be grouped together with some common property. For example, my water bottle and black stapler are both on my desk currently. I can artificially group them together and call them "watplers," which are either water bottles or black staplers. Although it is a fact about the world that there are two watplers on my desk, watplers is not a natural kind: they do not have any meaningful common properties. The tricky part is to figure out exactly what one means by "meaningful" properties. When we think about what the world consists of, if there were no one around, we do not think of watplers. They are too artificial and too arbitrarily grouped together to be considered things that are "naturally" in the world, so to speak.

We can think of conditions (2) and (3) as attempts to clarify our intuition about what constitutes a meaningful property. These two conditions trade on the presupposition that natural kinds are like nodes in the structure of universe. Many of us believe that things and events in nature do not behave or occur independently of one another. The drinking of a large quantity of arsenic, for instance, led to, caused, or necessitated (in philosophical jargon) the death of the person who drank it. The drinking and the subsequent death are not independent or isolated events. Likewise, when I strike a cue ball and it hits the 8 ball which then rolls into the corner pocket, these events are not random. The laws of physics dictate that the 8 ball *must* roll into the pocket (all else being equal).[10] Likewise, $E = mc^2$ does not merely mean that, as a matter of contingent fact, the amounts of energy of a body *happens* to be the same as its mass multiplied by the speed of light squared; rather, the energy of a body *must* be equal to that amount. This kind of metaphysical necessity is indispensable if we view the universe as consisting of not merely isolated events, but events that are linked to one another by some necessity. Scientific laws are attempts to understand the idea that the universe is structured in this sense. Natural kinds are special, according to some philosophers, because they alone can participate in the laws of nature. In other words, laws of nature relate the necessitation between natural kinds and natural kinds only.

One of the most celebrated arguments in recent history in favor of the existence of natural kinds comes from the work of the philosopher Hilary Putnam. In his oft-cited paper "The Meaning of Meaning" (1975), Putnam argues that terms like "water" function as natural kind terms. Their meaning is not dependent on our commonsensical understanding of them; rather, they are solely dependent on their micro-physical properties. In the case of a substance like water, Putnam argues that the term "water" refers to its atomic structure.

Suppose we are ignorant of the physical structure of water. Instead, we think of water as a colorless and odorless liquid that falls from the sky when it rains, fills our lakes and rivers, quenches our thirst, and so on. We might come to believe that the term "water" refers to a liquid that has these superficial characteristics. Suppose further that we travel to a Twin Earth that is almost identical to ours. It too has rain, rivers, and lakes filled with a colorless and odorless liquid. Twin People who live on Twin Earth also drink this liquid when they feel thirsty, swim in lakes filled with it, and shower with this stuff coming out of their showerheads. Advances in chemistry on Earth discover that the colorless and odorless liquid that we call "water" back home is in fact made up of H_2O and, amazingly, the corresponding liquid on Twin Earth that functions just like our water is made up of an entirely exotic material XYZ. Our intuition is that their "water" is in fact not water, because what makes water water is the underlying atomic structure and not its superficial characteristics and functions. We would not say that Twin Earth has water and that its water is made of XYZ; rather, we would say that Twin Earth has this stuff that looks and behaves a lot like our water but it is not water because it is made of XYZ. If "water" just means colorless odorless liquid that falls from the sky and quenches our thirst, then Twin Water should be called "water." The fact that we intuitively do not believe Twin Water is water tells us that "water" picks out some deep atomic structure.

This is so even if we were entirely unaware of this structure or even the theory of identifying physical substances with their atomic structures. One way to explain the objectivity of terms like "water," "gold," and "electrons" is that these terms pick out real categories of things in the world; they pick out natural kinds. Twin Earth might have sandwiches, but if we discover that they are not made of the same physical stuff as ours, we would not say they do not have sandwiches. We would instead say their sandwiches are made of more exotic stuff. The different intuitions we have towards water and sandwiches are because the former is a natural kind and the latter is not.

One can see how a naturalist might be drawn to the concept of natural kinds because they provide a convenient basis on which a naturalist might be able to define disease and health in terms of objective categories. Take cholera as an example. Before discovering that cholera is caused by infections from *Vibrio cholerae* bacterium, physicians thought that it was the body's response to excess bile that itself was caused by a choleric personality. The vomiting and diarrhea that are symptomatic of cholera, they believed, were the body's attempt to purge the excessive bile. The discovery of a bacterial cause to cholera did not lead physicians to conclude that there was no cholera after all. In contrast, physicians re-identified cholera with its underlying pathology. Natural kinds offer a conceptual framework to justify the identification of, say, disease with objective physical dysfunctions. And like the identification of water with H_2O, the identification of cholera with *Vibrio cholerae* bacterium's infection is an objective and value-neutral practice, or so the naturalists would like to think.

Whether we think there are actually natural kinds or not is less important for us than the immediate question of whether diseases (and health) are natural kinds.[11] There are two ways to understand this question. Is the general concept of a disease a natural kind? Alternatively, we might ask whether a *specific* disease is identical to some natural kind? Lawrie Reznek has argued persuasively that we should answer negatively to the first question.[12] His argument is straightforward. We often decide that certain physiological conditions are disease states well before the underlying physiological causes are identified. We consider depression a mental illness even though we have no clear understanding of the physiological causal pathway that gives rise to depression.

Moreover, we continue to maintain that a condition is a disease even if its underlying physical pathology does not fit well with the type of underlying pathology that we think diseases in general have. For instance, suppose we consider condition X a disease. And suppose we believe that all diseases and disorders pick out physiological functions that deviate from normal species functioning, as defined evolutionarily. If it turns out that having X does not conflict with any normal species functioning, we ought to conclude that X is not a disease, regardless of how X affects the life of a person with X. Yet, whether we want to maintain that X is a disease seems to be an open question. We might instead think that our belief that a disease picks out deviation from normal species functioning is wrong and that we need to do more work to find the real common underlying physiology that all diseases share. If, at the end of our search, there is no such common underlying physiology, we do not conclude that there are no diseases after all. We say instead that there are diseases, but that they don't have anything physiological in common. This tells us that disease and disorder, as broad concepts, are not natural kinds.

As to whether a *specific* disease is identical to some natural kind, the practice of clinical diagnoses seems to say otherwise as well. Take the broad diagnosis of cancer. We know that the etiology of cancer consists of a diverse range of possible suspects from genetic mutations at birth to exposures to environmental toxins, from the body's declining ability to repair cells to viral infections. It seems highly unlikely that there is one clear type of underlying physiological dysfunction that is responsible for cancer. Cancer is a remarkably broad diagnostic category that, in time, will likely be refined; for instance, conditions that we now think are cancerous might turn out not to be and vice versa. Nevertheless, the classifications of diseases often involve the grouping of widely diverse underlying causes that do not form any obvious natural kind.

Take focal segmental glomerulosclerosis (FSGS)—a disease categorized by the scarring of kidney tissues that can lead to kidney failures in adults and nephrotic syndrome in children. The causes for FSGS include obesity, lupus, heroin usage, and HIV. Primary FSGS is categorized as an idiopathic condition with unknown causes. FSGS represents a counter-example to those who define disease in terms of natural kinds. Not only are there no obvious natural kinds that underpin FSGS, the idiopathic variant (a common variation for many diseases) shows that diseases are sometimes grouped in terms of surface presentations that do not obviously share any common type of underlying pathologies and causes.

Philosophers often cite the gem jade as an example of a non-natural kind. It turns out that "jade" does not identify gems of a common molecular structure. There are in fact two different kinds of gems that we consider jade: jadeite ($NaAlSi_2O_6$) and nephrite ($Ca_2(Mg, Fe)_5Si_8O_{22}(OH)_2$). Although the two types of jade often appear similar, they are radically different chemically. The heterogeneous nature of jade disqualifies it from being a natural kind. But instead of saying jade does not exist upon the discovery of its twin molecular bases, we say that jade exists but it is not a natural kind. The heterogeneity of many disease states (everything from cancer to depression) perhaps warrants a similar conclusion. The multitude of pathologies when it comes to depression should not automatically lead us to conclude that there is no depression, but that depression turns out not to be a natural kind. The result tells us that specific diseases need not map neatly onto any common underlying natural kinds in order to be considered diseases.

2.5 Twin Goals of Medicine and Twin Definitions of Health

Both normativism and naturalism fail to capture all of our pre-theoretical intuitions, and exactly how much of this should affect the plausibility of their theories depends on how much we think a correct analysis of disease and health should capture our common usages. There is a hidden point of contention here that might help us understand the orientation of normativism vs. naturalism. Recall our discussion in the first chapter about the multiple goals of medicine. In addition to clinical and therapeutic practices that strive to improve our well-being, medicine is also a scientific endeavor that aims to contribute to our empirical knowledge (e.g., about human physiology and biology). The division between normativism and naturalism echoes this dichotomy. If medicine cares only about improving our well-being via medical means, then whether disease and health are ultimately grounded in some value-free objective fact becomes far less relevant. Some of the philosophical motivation behind normativism, I suspect, stems from a more basic belief that the primary aims of medicine center around its practical impacts on our well-being.

On the other hand, if we focus on medicine as a scientific pursuit akin to other scientific disciplines or sub-fields (e.g., astrophysics or evolutionary biology), we might want to ground concepts like disease and health on some objective empirical processes. In science, when something deviates from its normal behaviors, it does not necessarily mean it is a bad thing from our point of view. Most materials contract when cooled. Water is a remarkable exception: it expands when it becomes solid. This "abnormality" is morally neutral. Indeed, one might even say that it is fortuitous for us that water deviates from the usual behaviors of physical substances. The fact that ice is less dense than liquid water, for instance, allows ice to float, creating a thermal insulation on the surface of lakes and rivers. This layer prevents large bodies of water from entirely freezing over, thus allowing many aquatic organisms (including our ancestors) to survive during cold winters. Medicine as science can view health and disease along these same lines.

The two goals of medicine are certainly not independent of one another. One of the reasons why the discoveries of regularities and laws in medicine are so important is that they allow us to confidently practice clinical care. Cutting smoking lowers one's risks for cardiovascular diseases. This is not just a matter of coincidence or accident; this is a matter of objective causal relationships grounded in the laws of nature. How we integrate and translate these two parts of medicine with their different understandings of disease and health is an important question that carries significant ethical weight. Real lives are at stake. In medical ethics, we have the domain of translational ethics in which theorists address challenges that confront medicine when we attempt to apply results from research medicine to clinical practices. Many of these difficulties, it might turn out, stem from the twin goals of medicine and their different understandings of disease and health.

Notes

1 The birthplace of Spam—Austin, Minnesota—launched an autism-friendly movement in 2008. The town offers workshops to teach business owners how to accommodate the needs of autists such as lowering the level of noise and visual stimulations. The effort proved so successful that families with autistic members moved to Austin for the town's sensibility.

2 Of course, a condition not being a disability does not automatically mean that one is not entitled to political and social support. If there is widespread discrimination against individuals with a certain religious affiliation, one is entitled to protection. In the case of autism, whether we construe it as a disease or not does not definitively settle the question of autists' rights to accommodations.

3 We will put aside the concern that scientific facts are objective and value-free things for the moment. In Chapter 3 and Chapter 7, we will examine this claim more closely.

4 The idea that we can clearly identify the evolutionary purposes of any biological trait is by no means uncontroversial. Consider the evolutionary path that (head) hair took. Presumably, hair offered a great deal of evolutionary benefits because it kept our ancestors warm. The thermal advantage of hair is far less important in modern societies where hats are available. Yet, suppose that having a rich head full of hair is considered attractive, thus granting the hairy individual an advantage in reproduction. Is the evolutionary purpose of hair insulation or mating? Whether a genotype is evolutionarily advantageous depends on its phenotypical effects on the genes' reproductive fitness and the latter is relative to the environment. What is advantageous in one context might be a costly mutation in another.

5 When philosophers attempt to explicate a concept, they often begin with clear positive instances of the concept and clear negative ones. The task is to figure out what those positive instances have in common and create a theory that might link them together and sharpen the boundary between the positive and negative instances. It is possible that after a careful analysis, it turns out that our pre-theoretical usages of the concept were completely mistaken. When this happens, it is imperative that one offers an explanation as to why we were so utterly wrong. The reason is that without an account that explains away the errors of our ways, the analysis might have replaced the concept that prompted our initial investigation with a new artificial one. Instead of providing an explication, one has merely changed the subject.

6 The idea that homosexuality can have an underlying physiology is not entirely beyond the realm of medical possibility. In 2017, Bogaert et al. published a paper in *The Proceedings of the National Academy of Science of the United States* in which they claim that a maternal immune response during male fetal brain development offers a possible explanation for why gay men, on average, have more older brothers.

7 George Williams' classic paper, "Pleiotropy, Natural Selection, and the Evolution of Senescence" (1957), offers just such a hypothesis.
8 It is important to remember that genes do not intend to do anything, nor do they have any agendas or purposes. The use of these terms is purely metaphorical and they merely are placeholders for a less picturesque and less teleological way of talking about natural selection.
9 For an in-depth discussion of the ways transposons might transmit horizontally from one organism to another, see Silva, Loreto, and Clark (2004). It is a rather technical paper but there is still a great deal of information to glean, even for those not well-versed in genetics.
10 The careful reader might notice that "all else being equal" is doing a great deal of work here. To say that the 8 ball will roll into the corner pocket, all else being equal, is to say that unless something unusual happens and the 8 ball is prevented from rolling into the pocket, it would do so. This is akin to asserting the tautology that the 8 ball will roll into the pocket unless it doesn't. Attempts to spell out exactly what "all else being equal" means have proven to be remarkably challenging. There seems to be no way to explicate it without rendering the claim trivially true.
11 The philosopher Tyler Burge (1979) famously argued that one can extend the kind of Twin Earth argument to generate similar intuitions about diseases like arthritis.
12 See Reznek (1995), for example.

References

Bogaert, A. F., Skorska, M. N., Wang, C., Gabrie, J., MacNeil, A. J., Hoffarth, M. R., . . . Blanchard, R. (2017). Male homosexuality and maternal immune responsivity to the y-linked protein NLGN4Y. *Proceedings of the National Academy of Sciences*. doi:10.1073/pnas.1705895114

Boorse, C. (1997). A rebuttal on health. In J. M. Humber & R. F. Almeder (Eds.), *What is disease?* (pp. 1–134). Totowa, NJ: Humana Press.

Burge, T. (1979). Individualism and the mental. *Midwest Studies in Philosophy*, *4*(1), 73–122.

Cooper, R. (2002). Disease. *Studies in History and Philosophy of Science Part C: Studies in History and Philosophy of Biological and Biomedical Sciences*, *33*(2), 263–282.

Daniels, N. (2000). Normal functioning and the treatment-enhancement distinction. *Cambridge Quarterly of Healthcare Ethics*, *9*(3), 309–322.

Downie, J. A. (2005). Legume haemoglobins: Symbiotic nitrogen fixation needs bloody nodules. *Current Biology*, *15*(6), R196–R198. doi:https://doi.org/10.1016/j.cub.2005.03.007

Granville, J. M. (1883). *Nerve-vibration and excitation as agents in the treatment of functional disorder and organic disease*. London: J. & A. Churchill.

Graur, D. (2015). *Molecular and genome evolution*. Sunderland, MA: Sinauer.

National Symposium on Neurodiversity. (2011). *Statement on Neurodiversity*. https://neurodiversitysymposium.wordpress.com. Accessed 3/30/2019.

Oliveira, S. G., Bao, W., Martins, C., & Jurka, J. (2012). Horizontal transfers of mariner transposons between mammals and insects. *Mobile DNA*, *3*(1), 14. doi:10.1186/1759-8753-3-14

Putnam, H. (1975). The meaning of "Meaning". *Minnesota Studies in the Philosophy of Science*, 7, 131–193.

Reznek, L. (1995). Dis-ease about kinds: Reply to D'amico. *Journal of Medicine and Philosophy*, *20*(5), 571–584. doi:10.1093/jmp/20.5.571

Silva, J. C., Loreto, E. L., & Clark, J. B. (2004). Factors that affect the horizontal transfer of transposable elements. *Current Issues in Molecular Biology*, *6*(1), 57–71.

Struchiner, C. J., Kidwell, M. G., & Ribeiro, J. M. C. (2005). Population dynamics of transposable elements: Copy number regulation and species invasion requirements. *Journal of Biological Systems, 13*(04), 455–475. doi:10.1142/s021833900500163x

Tawakol, A., Ishai, A., Takx, R. A. P., Figueroa, A. L., Ali, A., Kaiser, Y., . . . Pitman, R. K. (2017). Relation between resting amygdalar activity and cardiovascular events: A longitudinal and cohort study. *The Lancet, 389*(10071), 834–845. doi:10.1016/S0140-6736(16)31714-7

Williams, G. C. (1957). Pleiotropy, natural selection, and the evolution of senescence. *Evolution, 11*(4), 398–411. doi:10.2307/2406060

3

EVIDENCE IN MEDICINE

3.1 Getting It Right for the Right Reasons

The importance of evidence in any pursuit of knowledge is obvious. Having merely true beliefs is typically not sufficient for knowledge. For instance, suppose I guessed that you were born on June 24 and suppose that you *were* indeed born on June 24. No ordinary understanding of knowledge would consider my correct guess as being knowledge. If I consistently guess right, there might be some use for my talents (and we might even explore deeper just exactly *how* I am so good at making birthday guesses). But, from an epistemic point of view, my correct guess was just so much sheer luck.

When it comes to medical research and clinical practice, we want to not merely get it right; we want to get it right for the right reason. The reasons that support our beliefs represent the epistemic foundation; they elevate mere guesses to something better, such as justified beliefs. We will use the phrase "epistemic virtues" to refer to features of our beliefs that render them better from an epistemic point of view. Think in terms of the difference between beliefs that are well-supported by evidence and reasons and beliefs that are not. The purpose of this chapter is to explore broadly the idea of epistemic virtue; that is, what distinguishes mere opinions and correct guesses from justified beliefs and knowledge?

Philosophers have thought about the nature of knowledge, justification, certainty, and other epistemic virtues for millennia. But unlike some purely abstract philosophical questions, epistemology can have a great deal at stake. All things being equal, we *ought* to act on the basis of beliefs that are epistemically superior. The need to be on sound epistemic footing becomes even more urgent when someone's life or life-prospect depends on it. We want our medicine properly grounded, because without some reason to think our medical beliefs are true, we would have little confidence in thinking that diagnoses and therapeutic judgments are appropriate. We might just have gotten really lucky with past correct proclamations. In some respects, our basic commitment to ethical medicine requires that we act upon the best available medical knowledge. To do otherwise is to be negligent. Thus, knowing what constitutes evidence and medical knowledge is a *moral* imperative.

The recent emergence of Evidence-Based Medicine—as an epistemic and professional movement—reflects, I believe, some of this moral impetus. As soon as we realize that evidence and epistemic virtues come in different types and grades, it becomes critical that we understand the strengths and weaknesses of each type of epistemic support. Is anecdotal evidence better than extrapolating therapeutic recommendations from our understanding of physiology and pharmacokinetics? Should we refrain from funding exotic research projects (such as one that studies the therapeutic benefits of intercessory prayers) because they conflict with our well-confirmed understanding of physiology and naturalism in general?

In addition to a renewed commitment to ground medical practice in the best evidence, medical research is arguably at a moment of self-reflection. The "Replication Crisis" continues to identify classic experiments and results, ranging from psychology to oncology, that we cannot replicate.[1] Add to that revelations of data fudging and fraud (George & Buyse, 2015), *p*-hacking (a research practice that we will explore later in this chapter), and the frustratingly frequent reversals of medical recommendations (e.g., is coffee bad for you?), it is no wonder that many people's confidence in medicine is waning. In order to restore and nurture trust in medicine, we must ensure that research and clinical medicine sit on a firm epistemic foundation. At the very least, we ought to sort out what we know, what we don't know, and the boundaries of what we can know.

This discussion in this chapter is divided into two sections. In the first, we will discuss some deep and recalcitrant problems with the use of evidence in our orthodox model of experimental science; specifically, how does an observation provide evidence to support a hypothesis? Some of the issues might appear abstract, but they will help reveal the limits and nature of evidential reasoning (i.e., using evidence to reason). Realizing what we are entitled to assert on the basis of the evidence would go a long way to steer medicine onto a clearer epistemic path. In the second section, we will focus on some of the more practical issues that challenge the production of medical knowledge. Although less philosophical, these problems reveal some deep concerns about how we can have a sound method of science amidst our social institutions and forces. Perhaps some of the epistemic problems with medicine such as the Replication Crisis are bigger than just age-old philosophical difficulties rearing their ugly heads; they might be the products of, or exacerbated by, the social, political, and economic contexts that surround medicine. To "fix" medicine, we might have to change the structure of our society.

The philosophical issues with regards to the use of evidence are also connected to how we understand scientific explanations and probability. For example, when a physician attempts to identify the likely cause of a patient's symptoms, she gathers evidence (e.g., blood work, vital signs, patient's reports, etc.) and infers a specific diagnosis that best explains the evidence. Similarly, some philosophers take an observation to be evidence for a hypothesis if it raises the probability of the hypothesis. The three concepts of evidence, explanation, and probability are deeply intertwined. After taking a closer look at the nature of evidence, we will turn to explanation and probability in the next two chapters.

3.2 The Story of Adelina

Many years ago, I met an elderly Italian woman, Adelina, in Rome who lived in an apartment next door to a dear friend. Her unassuming appearance would not give any hint of her celebrity status among the locals. In addition to her father being the mason who restored the beloved bell tower of San Marco in Venice (where they would invite her as the guest of honor for an annual parade), she also interpreted x-rays sent to her from hospitals across Italy and the world. She showed me letters of gratitude from hospitals for her service. Apparently, she was remarkably good at detecting pathologies revealed by the x-rays. As far as I know, she never received any training in radiography and, short of a vague instinct, she could not explain how she was able to perform the task so accurately.[2]

When Adelina says, "This patient has cancer," we do not think that Adelina *knows* that the patient has cancer. She might be correct, even repeatedly so, but having a true belief is not sufficient for knowledge. After all, she might have been merely lucky (albeit, more incredibly so with each correct reading). For us to be convinced that she knows, we need to understand *how* she is getting it right so often. Suppose we discover later that she is able to discern from the x-rays some fuzzy images of enzymes that only certain cancer cells produce. Perhaps Adelina is entirely unaware of her ability to spot these enzymes and her cancer predictions are (unconsciously) dependent on detecting their presence. If we could find such a link, we might conclude that Adelina does in fact know the presence of cancer by looking at those x-rays. We (and she) simply didn't understand how she does it. Contrary to the appearance, there is, in fact, a method to the madness.

The precise nature of the additional condition that must be satisfied to turn true beliefs into knowledge is an ongoing and lively debate in philosophy. For our purpose, however, we will take a broader view. Rather than focusing on what constitutes knowledge per se, we can instead think about what makes something "epistemically superior" or "epistemically more virtuous." In general, we think that some beliefs are epistemically superior to other beliefs. For instance, suppose I believe that Sandra's favorite color is blue and Aisha's is brown. Suppose I hold the former belief because Sandra has told me so. In the case of Aisha, however, I leapt to the conclusion because I saw Aisha wear a brown sweater once. All else being equal, the former opinion is epistemically better grounded or justified than the latter. The philosophical question before us is what makes some beliefs epistemically superior in this broad sense?

3.3 Confirming Hypotheses With Evidence

One way we can explain why a belief is epistemically superior to another is by noting the evidential difference between the two; for example, a belief is epistemically superior if it has greater evidential support than another. Of course, evidence and evidential support are not binary concepts; they come in grades across a variety of vectors. They can differ in both quality and quantity. Anecdotal evidence or a clinician's past experience, for instance, provides *some* support for the recommendation of a particular treatment. Indeed, one could have an abundance of anecdotal evidence that a treatment is therapeutically beneficial. However, we might learn from randomized double-blind control trials that the treatment, in fact, provides very few benefits. Here, the evidential quality of clinical trials might trump the support provided by a plethora of personal testimony and clinical experience.

Similarly, certain treatments can also become standard care because of commonsense expectations. The recommendation of surgery (debulking) to remove as many cancer cells as possible before chemotherapy or radiation treatment seems reasonable. After all, why zap cancer cells when one could remove them en masse physically and let chemotherapy and radiation do the mopping up? As compelling as this narrative appears, it turned out that surgical debulking might provide very few additional therapeutic benefits for certain cancers (Schorge, McCann, & Del Carmen, 2010). Here, the epistemic strength of clinical trials seems to overturn years of accepted practice, anecdotal evidence, and bio-plausibility—a term used to refer to physiologically reasonable treatments.

In ordinary usage, the term "evidence" includes a wide range of usages. The yellowing of the sclerae of the eyes is evidence that an individual might have jaundice. A randomized clinical trial offers evidence that a treatment is therapeutically beneficial. A clinician's past experience provides anecdotal evidence that a chemotherapy regimen is a promising off-label treatment for some forms of cancer. The concept of evidence here includes signs for illnesses, research justifications for therapeutic protocols, and rationales for clinical decisions. A unified theory of medical evidence would clearly be beyond the scope of this chapter (or book!). But, we can still say something meaningful about the nature of evidence in medicine.

One of the basic beliefs about evidence is that, all else being equal, it increases our confidence in the claim that the evidence aims to support. Noticing the yellowness in one's sclerae increases our confidence that the person has jaundice. Likewise, clinical studies can supply evidence that increases our confidence in the therapeutic benefit of a treatment. In fact, this relationship between evidence and its ability to increase our confidence borders on being true by definition: some philosophers have defined the concept of evidence in terms of its ability to raise the subjective probability (a measurement of confidence) of a hypothesis. Formally, one might say that

$$\text{E is evidence for H} \equiv P(H/E) > P(H)$$

Or, less formally, E is a piece of evidence for the hypothesis H if and only if the probability of the hypothesis H given E is greater than the probability of H by itself. This definition, of course, does not tell us *if* and *how* a given piece of evidence increases the probability of a hypothesis. It only says that for something to qualify as evidence, it ought to increase the probability of the hypothesis that it aims to support. This view seems reasonable enough; after all, it would be odd to say that E is evidence for H but learning about E actually *lowers* our confidence that H is true.

Not all positive instances qualify as supporting evidence for a hypothesis. The American philosopher Nelson Goodman has written extensively on the difference.[3] Consider the generalization "All emeralds are green." Finding a particular green emerald (a positive instance) seems to provide confirming evidence for the generalization "All emeralds are green." As a scientific law, "All emeralds are green" is not just a description of the brute reality of the universe (that is, as a matter of contingent fact, all emeralds *happen* to be green). Rather, the generalization is usually taken to convey certain necessity. Emeralds, by virtue of what they are, *must* be green. This kind of necessity is often referred to as nomological necessity or necessity based on some laws of nature. To put it in terms of the schema we mentioned before, we can say that P (all emeralds are green/a particular green emerald) > P (all emeralds are green); that is, the observation of a particular green emerald is evidence for the hypothesis that all emeralds are green because it raises the probability that the law is true. In this sense, amassing positive instances provides growing evidential support for a hypothesis, and that is the reason why a larger sample offers greater evidential support. To be sure, no amount of finite positive instances can guarantee that the hypothesis is true. The possibility remains that we can come across a negative instance that would undermine our hypothesis. Finding an emerald that is purple, for example, would surely shake our confidence that all emeralds are green.

When a positive instance raises the probability of a hypothesis, we say the hypothesis is further confirmed. The possibility of a counter-example makes it impossible for us to *guarantee* the truth of a hypothesis in light of finite evidence. In this sense, one can never "prove" the truth of a scientific claim by appealing to evidence (if "prove" means logically guarantee). Likewise, one cannot prove a negation or absence of something empirically. Unless we have searched every corner of the universe, it would be impossible to guarantee that unicorns do not exist. But this presents no unique epistemic challenge. For instance, we have a great deal of evidence that the extra chromosome 21 causes Down syndrome; yet it is entirely possible that the cause is indeed something else. Our belief that a third chromosome 21 causes Down syndrome is well confirmed, but not logically guaranteed. We can no more "prove" the non-existence of unicorns than we can "prove" that the presence of a third chromosome 21 causes Down syndrome. In empirical confirmation, a hypothesis is confirmed as a matter of degree ranging exclusively from 0 or 1. In order to accept a scientific hypothesis, we do not need to guarantee that it is true; we only need to have sufficient confirmation of its truth.

Consider, however, the following exceptionless regularity (a regularity without any counter-examples): all residents of China are under 120 years old. As a matter of fact, this is true. (If doubts creep in, we can jack up the age to make it more plausible.) But, this regularity does not afford confirmation akin to the generalization that all emeralds are green. The tallying of yet another Chinese resident who is less than 120 years old does not strengthen our confidence that it is a law of nature that Chinese residents cannot be over 120. There is nothing nomologically necessary between being a resident of China and being under 120. After all, it is logically, if not biologically, possible that someone in China lives beyond 120 years. This individual would not simply go out of existence on his birthday just because he was living in China as he turned 120. For this reason, Goodman (1983) argues that whether a hypothesis can be confirmed by evidence depends on more than just the logical structure of the inductive argument. Finding an instance of X that is a Y does not automatically mean that there is evidential support for the hypothesis "All Xs are Ys." We need to know something about the content of the hypothesis (the nature of the X and Y) to determine whether the hypothesis is something that can be confirmed. Goodman says that concepts like "green" and "emeralds" are projectable and that generalizations that contain them are capable of being confirmed. "Being a resident of China" and "being less that 120 years old" are not projectable.

3.4 Projectability

For Goodman, what distinguishes projectable concepts and non-projectable ones is not intrinsic to the concepts themselves. His "gruebleen" example, which is arguably one of the most well-known examples in 20th century philosophy, illustrates the argument (Goodman, 1983). Consider the regularity "All emeralds are grue." "Grue" is an entirely made-up concept and it is defined as something that is green and observed before, say, the year 2050 or is blue otherwise. Every emerald that we have observed is green, but it is also true that every emerald we have observed is grue (since it was observed before 2050 and was green). Suppose we are on the eve of 2050. What should we say about the emeralds we find tomorrow? According to the hypothesis "All emeralds are green," we should expect the emeralds we examine for the first-time tomorrow to be green. However, according to the equally well-confirmed hypothesis "All emeralds are grue," we should expect to find emeralds that are blue.[4] Which hypothesis should we accept? Which prediction should we have confidence in? Or to put the question more philosophically, why do we think that "green" is projectable and "grue" not?

Responses to Goodman's argument (also known as the New Problem of Induction) have largely failed to identify properties that would justify our reliance

FIGURE 3.1 Gred

A sample of gred, which is a color that is observed before 2030 and is gray or otherwise red. If, after 2030, a reader finds this not to be red and this patch has not been previously observed, then obviously the wrong color was printed.

on green over grue. For instance, one might suggest that "grue" has a built-in temporal component (i.e., the year 2050) and that alone disqualifies it for being projectable. There are two problems with this response. First, one needs an additional argument as to why containing a temporal element renders a concept non-projectable. It might be true that projectable concepts cannot contain references to the Gregorian calendar, but we should not simply assume this. Secondly, Goodman argues that whether "grue" contains a temporal element depends upon certain historic contingencies. If we define "grue" in terms of green and blue, then we would need to add the temporal qualifier. However, if we define "green" in terms of "grue" and "bleen" (defined as something that is blue and observed before 2050 or green otherwise), then it is "blue" and "green" that contain temporal references. The concept "green" defined with "grue" and "bleen" would thus be a color that is grue and observed before year 2050 or bleen afterwards. In this alternate history, it is "green" and "blue" that contain temporal references and not "grue" and "bleen!" Goodman concludes that there is nothing inherently special about predicates like "blue" and "green." They *seem* projectable only because they are more entrenched; that is, we started using them early on and we built a host of theories and worldviews on top of them. To insist that "green" is nomologically special and "grue" is not is to use seniority and historic contingencies as the marks of metaphysical significance.

Goodman's observation that projectability is a result of contingent historic choices entails consequences that are relevant to the use of evidence in medicine. For starters, the claim that certain concepts are not projectable, and hence no positive instances can confirm generalizations containing them, rests on rather shaky grounds. If projectability depends on an historical accident of which concepts came first and got entrenched, then whether a hypothesis can be confirmed also depends on these historical contingencies. For those who believe that laws reveal the real nomological structure of the universe, this would certainly be a disappointing result. If Goodman is right, laws of nature are merely regularities that we happen to treat as laws; they pick out nothing metaphysically deep about the world.

Goodman's argument goes beyond challenging a meaningful division between projectable and non-projectable concepts. His argument also shows that a blanket dismissal of empirical research into exotic hypotheses (e.g., astrological impacts on health outcomes) is likely unwarranted. An opponent of exotic hypotheses might suggest that no matter how much evidence researchers have collected, if the terms in these hypotheses are not projectable, these hypotheses cannot be supported by evidence. Amassing a volume of instances of Geminis who develop type-2 diabetes, they argue, would not add any evidential support for the hypothesis that Geminis are more likely to develop type-2 diabetes. Being a Gemini is not the sort of thing that can be projectable or can participate in laws of nature. However, if projectability turns out to be a rather philosophically trivial concept, then a rejection of exotic research projects on the grounds that it contains non-projectable terms would lack serious philosophical justification.

When a particular concept becomes entrenched as a projectable, it sets up constraints on whether a new term is projectable or not. Suppose we decide that "emerald" is a projectable term. We might look to the stable crystalline structures of emeralds as the *reason* to justify or to explain its projectability. This connection helps form a metaphysical view of the world. As we continue to do science and to categorize terms as projectable, these decisions help weave together a picture of how the universe works. Moreover, this emerging and deep metaphysical picture of the world helps dictate the direction of future research. For instance, if we accept (implicitly or otherwise) the idea that microscopic structural properties can affect macroscopic observations, then a hypothesis that rejects this connection would likely be considered not projectable (and hence not a part of any scientific laws).

We can explain our inclination to reject certain observations as evidence for confirming exotic hypotheses along this line. It just seems crazy to think that the retrograde motion of Mercury, which is the result of relative motions between Earth and Mercury, has anything to do with our physiological and psychological well-being. How can an optical illusion affect my health? It simply does not fit into our metaphysical picture of the way the world is, as woven together by generations of past decisions about projectability.

Take for instance the use of intercessory prayers to improve clinical outcomes. Leonard Leibovici (2001) published a spoof that showed that patients with a bloodstream infection in a double-blind controlled trial who were being prayed for, unbeknownst to them, had statistically better outcomes. Leibovici's piece, indeed, went one step farther: not only were prayers therapeutically effective for living patients, prayers improved health outcomes of patients who had long died! His intention was to demonstrate that one can use data in accordance with the standards of scientific rigor to support ridiculous hypotheses. Many readers did not know of his hidden agenda, and the idea that prayers could work post-mortem was just a bridge too far; Leibovici's paper was met with laughter, confusion, and demands that the British Medical Journal retract it.

But what exactly is so ridiculous about the results? Why do these positive instances not count as evidence for the therapeutic benefits of remote retroactive intercessory prayers? His conclusion is ridiculous because it violates some of our deeply held beliefs about the way the world is. The causal power of supernatural prayers, which are, by definition, beyond the natural, conflicts with our metaphysical assumption that causality must involve interactions between physical things. The number 4, for instance, cannot trip you as you walk down the street because it is an abstract entity unable to interact causally with physical things. Moreover, we believe that causality is temporally directional; that is, when A causes B, then A must precede B. One cannot cause something in the past, so to speak.[5] It borders on incoherence to say that we could pray for someone's health and the prayer would somehow go back in time to improve the health of a patient who has already died. Leibovici's joke precisely takes advantage of the incongruity between the alleged therapeutic pathway of retroactive intercessory prayers and everything we (implicitly or explicitly) believe about how our bodies (and causation in general) work. Without a plausible narrative that fits the causal power of intercessory prayers into our metaphysical worldview, prayers cannot be projectable. In this respect, no amount of positive instances can serve as evidential confirmation for the therapeutic benefits of prayers. The practice of science, including judging whether a hypothesis is opened to evidential support, requires practitioners to make certain metaphysical assumptions. Like it or not, scientists are always doing philosophy.

The present discussion is more than just of academic interest. Whether we deem something a legitimate or even plausible research project has many real-life consequences. No self-respecting scientific funding body, for example, would financially support a study that seeks to measure the weight of the human soul. Worse yet, clinicians might dismiss mountains of data that seemingly demonstrate the therapeutic benefits of an exotic treatment because "it just couldn't possibly work!" Scientists like to pride themselves as open-minded seekers of truths, however uncomfortable, unconventional, and counterintuitive these truths might be. In reality, exotic research approaches are often dismissed because they conflict with our preconceived ideas of the way the world is. As Thomas Kuhn points out, normal science is conservative, restrictive, and dogmatic. The metaphysical and epistemic rules of the prevailing paradigm not only tell us how to do science, they also often tell us emphatically what counts as science.

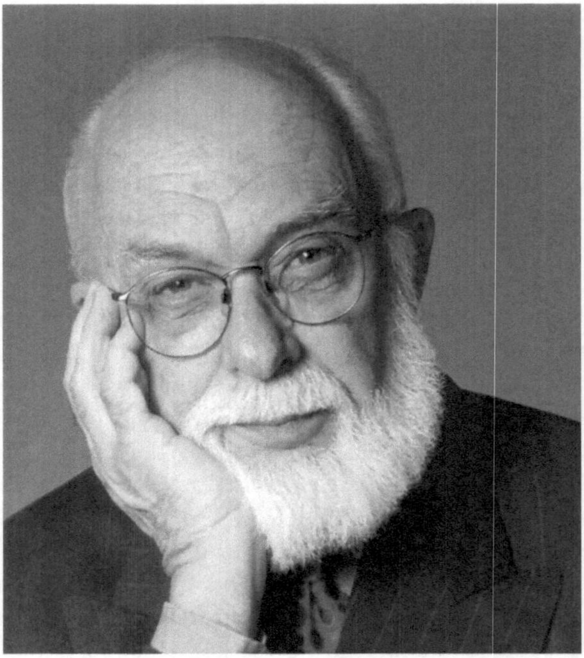

FIGURE 3.2 James Randi

James Randi, aka The Amazing Randi, spent the better part of his career debunking charlatans and scammers. Self-proclaimed faith healers were some of his favorite targets. Using his background as a professional magician, Randi unmasked the tricks they used to fool their victims. One of his most admirable qualities was that he did not dismiss claims of faith healing as impossible; instead, he treated them as empirical claims worthy of scientific investigations. For a superb documentary on his life and work, see *An Honest Liar. Source:* James Randi Educational Foundation, https://web.randi.org/.

3.5 Metaphysical Stories About the World

Projectability, law, and susceptibility to evidential support are deeply tied to the concept of plausible narrative. Very roughly, if we cannot tell a story of how one thing can affect another, we would remain skeptical that the statistical correlations between them are anything but coincidences. Notice that our use of "narrative" here is fairly vague. This is intentional. The idea is to leave enough conceptual space to accommodate a wide gamut of nomological connections. The nomological connection between two events can be causal, and it would account for how the occurrence of one (cause) necessitates another (effect). Understanding the nomological connection in terms of causality amounts to accepting a causal narrative of the metaphysical structure of the world. This narrative might have many gaps (e.g., we don't know exactly how causation works), but accepting it means that we see physically related events as causally related in a rough and ready sense. There is an implicit faith that the day will come when we can identify the causal pathway between events whose interaction currently remains unknown.

Of course, causality is just one of many possible ways we can understand how events in the world are connected. Consider a theistic example. The Red Sea parted because Moses raised his staff. One understanding of the relationship between the raising of Moses' staff and the parting of the Red Sea is that God intervened and pushed the waters apart. Divine interventions are not typically thought of as physical events. Yet, we want to say that Moses lifting his staff did lead to the parting of the sea with God doing much of the actual work. If we are to keep an open mind regarding the nomological connections of our universe, we ought to have a concept of narrative that does not preclude specific kinds of interaction.

Exotic nomological connections occur in the sciences as well. Since Newton's introduction of gravitational attraction (let alone since the ancient discovery of magnets), we have accepted the concept of actions at a distance; that is, objects can affect one another even if there is no physical contact between them. In 1935, Albert Einstein, Boris Podolsky, and Nathan Rosen offered a thought experiment in which, according to quantum mechanics, the measurement of one particle can affect the behavior of another particle. However, the only way this could happen is if the interaction travels faster than the speed of light. While Einstein et al. conclude that quantum mechanics does not provide a complete picture of the universe, many contemporary physicists accept the view that quantum mechanical interactions can consist of non-local actions at a distance. If we want to say that there is a nomological connection between these particles, then our metaphysical narrative of *how* this could happen must include interactions that go beyond our orthodox notion of causality.

Recent discussions of ontological grounding can help us illuminate and sketch out this basic concept of metaphysical connection between things in the world. The American philosopher Gideon Rosen, for instance, offers a concept of metaphysical dependency between events that include but are not exhausted by causation. Rosen, for instance, gives us this example:

> A glass is fragile in virtue of the arrangement of the molecules that make it up, perhaps together with the laws of chemistry and physics. One of the aims of materials science is to identify the physical bases of such dispositions.
> *(Rosen, 2010, p. 110)*

The molecular arrangement of glass does not *cause* its fragility in any ordinary sense of "cause," even though its molecular arrangement is *responsible* for its fragility. According to an orthodox understanding of causality, for event A to cause event B, A must precede B in time. The microscopic structure of glass does not precede its fragility. Likewise, we know that the molecular structure of sugar is responsible for its solubility. Yet, we do not want to say that its solubility is caused by its structure. When we discover the exact molecular properties that are responsible for solubility, we can make some generalizations about other substances and their degrees of solubility; e.g., we might be able to say that if X has a similar structure, it too would be soluble. This sort of nomological generalization is obviously not causal. Without an argument for treating causation as the only way things in the world can relate, we ought to have a concept of metaphysical narrative broad enough to include these non-causal dependencies. To insist otherwise is to make unwarranted metaphysical assumptions.

Dispositional properties like fragility and solubility are examples of non-causal dependencies. They illustrate a type of "vertical" dependency: macroscopic properties being dependent on microscopic properties. But there are "lateral" dependencies as well. Consider again the prayer example. Suppose that prayers actually improve the clinical outcomes of patients with blood infections. Suppose further that the "mechanism" by which prayers produce their therapeutic benefits is exactly as we think: God hears our prayers and divinely intervenes to improve patients' outcomes. Regardless of whether divine interventions are physical or causal relations, medicine and science at large would surely be interested in learning more about the interaction. To restrict our nomological narratives to include only causal relationships would automatically rule out any research in uncovering the non-causal nomological connection between prayers and health.

We can summarize the argument more explicitly this way:

(1) A positive instance is only evidence for a generalized hypothesis, if they contain projectable concepts.
(2) A concept is projectable only if it can be couched within a plausible nomological narrative that can explain *how* the interaction can take place.

Therefore, a positive instance is evidence for a hypothesis only if it can be couched within a plausible nomological narrative that can explain *how* the interaction can take place.

If we restrict nomological narratives to those that contain certain kinds of metaphysical dependency (e.g., causality), then it follows that confirmability of a hypothesis depends on whether the hypothesis fits with the same type of metaphysical dependency. This result raises a couple of interesting questions. For starters, if, as Goodman argues, projectability (and existence of a nomological narrative) is a matter of social conventions or historical contingencies, then whether something serves as evidence would also be a matter of social conventions or historic contingencies. This consequence certainly casts some doubt on the idea that certain exotic research projects (such as the therapeutic power of prayers) are off-limits because they are nonsense or unscientific in some fundamental sense.

Secondly, if science prides itself on being non-dogmatic or open-minded, then we must be open-minded about what constitutes an acceptable nomological narrative. In other words, we could see the world as structured in several different ways. Unless we can show that some structural narratives (say, physical causality) are warranted, it would be presumptuous to rule out other nomological narratives. To reject "nonsense" studies like the therapeutic power of prayer because they don't fit into our nomological narrative is to assume consensus and certainty about the metaphysical structure of the world when there are none.

3.6 Revisiting Experimental Holism

In Chapter 1, we discussed Karl Popper's falsifiability as a demarcation criterion, and we concluded that Popper's proposal failed. The primary reason is that falsifiability presents an account of the practice of science that fails on logical ground. The historic example of Urbain Le Verrier's and John Adams' discovery of Neptune shows that when an experimental observation conflicts with a prediction, a scientist often examines the auxiliary hypotheses that she assumed in deriving her prediction. The failure of a prediction can be the fault of a false hypothesis, or it could be any one of the secondary assumptions, including many practical ones (e.g., was I drunk when I derived these calculations?). It is this holistic nature of falsification that delivers the fatal blow to Popper's suggestion that a hypothesis' ability to be falsified makes it scientific. It turns out, no hypothesis can be falsified in isolation. Whenever we test a hypothesis against a prediction, we are always testing it along with a corpus of assumptions, many of which we are unaware of.

Just as falsifiability cannot be done in isolation, its companion confirmation also suffers the same fate. When a hypothesis is being confirmed in light of some positive instance or correct prediction, we are also confirming the hypothesis along with a host of auxiliary assumptions. Of course, unlike a false prediction where there is the presence of some unexpected result, a true prediction does not generate the same surprise. As a result, the presence of a confirming instance gives us a deceptive reason to believe that the hypothesis is correct, since the hypothesis gave us the right result. Nevertheless, the same type of scientific holism that we find in falsification also exists for confirmation. Hypotheses are never confirmed in isolation; only the corpus of hypotheses together with the auxiliary assumptions can be holistically confirmed by evidence.

One consequence of this type of experimental holism is that we can question the grounds we have for believing that correct predictions raise our confidence in the hypothesis being tested. It is logically possible that false hypotheses, together with other false auxiliary assumptions, generate true predictions. Historically, there have been a plethora of false scientific theories that gave us highly accurate predictions. The Ptolemaic geocentric view of the solar system, for instance, was far more accurate in predicting the locations of celestial bodies than the Copernican heliocentric challenger in its early days. For medium-sized objects, Newtonian mechanics continue to provide accurate predictions even though Special Relativity has shown that Newton's theories are false. The history of science is peppered with false theories that give us accurate predictions.

If we choose hypotheses by the accuracy of their predictions, then we could very well have accepted plenty of hypotheses that are false.[6] The apparent gap between experimental success and the truth of theory behooves us to be conservative with regards to the metaphysical and epistemic status of our scientific claims. We know that science and medicine in particular can be incredibly useful, but before we leap from their success to the conclusion that science and medicine provide a true picture of the world, we need to address a host of difficult philosophical questions including the ones outlined here.[7] The philosophical uncertainty between evidence and hypotheses should translate into a healthy degree of epistemic humility.

3.7 Evidence-Based Medicine: Philosophy in Practice

To see how a careful examination of evidence can affect the way we practice medicine, let's look at the debate surrounding Evidence-Based Medicine. As a movement that aims to improve clinical medicine, Evidence-Based Medicine (EBM) arguably grew out of the research done at McMaster University in Canada in the 1980s. Its central idea is:

> Evidence-based medicine de-emphasizes intuition, unsystematic clinical experience, and pathophysiologic rationale as sufficient grounds for clinical decision making and stresses the examination of evidence from clinical research. Evidence-based medicine requires new skills of the physician, including efficient literature searching and the application of formal rules of evidence evaluating the clinical literature.
>
> *(Guyatt et al., 1992, p. 2420)*

For proponents of EBM, not all evidence carried the same weight. Randomized clinical trials (RCT), for instance, represent the "gold standard" of evidence. Indeed, following the suggestion of EBM, the Scottish Intercollegiate Guidelines Network (Harbour & Miller, 2001) developed a ranking of evidence for the National Health Services of Scotland which goes as follows:

- 1++ High quality meta-analyses, systematic reviews of RCTs, or RCTs with a very low risk of bias
- 1+ Well conducted meta-analyses, systematic reviews of RCTs, or RCTs with a low risk of bias
- 1− Meta-analyses, systematic reviews or RCTs, or RCTs with a high risk of bias
- 2++ High quality systematic reviews of case-control or cohort studies or high quality case- control or cohort studies with a very low risk of confounding, bias, or chance and a high probability that the relationship is causal
- 2+ Well conducted case-control or cohort studies with a low risk of confounding, bias, or chance and a moderate probability that the relationship is causal
- 2− Case-control or cohort studies with a high risk of confounding, bias, or chance and a significant risk that the relationship is not causal

- 3 Non-analytic studies, e.g. case reports, case series
- 4 Expert opinion

Although the ranking makes explicit what the committee sees are the relative evidential merit of each kind of evidence, when it comes to adjudicating conflicting evidence (often from different levels), the committee does not provide any clear procedure of how one ought to move forward. In these situations, the committee recommends that clinicians exercise "judgment based on clinical experience as well as knowledge of the evidence and the method used to generate it." It is certainly worth reiterating the importance that sound evidence guides healthcare delivery; nonetheless, "exercise good sense (a la Duhem's suggestion)" might rob EBM of its significance and usefulness.

EBM has undergone many revisions since its introduction in the 1990s, but its veneration of RCTs continues. The British philosopher John Worrall (2007) raises a number of problems with assigning such heavy evidential weight to RCTs. Among them, one relates nicely to our discussion. Consider the importance of controlling for confounders in a RCT. Researchers attempt the best that they can to control for any factors that could explain away the statistical significance of an experimental results without attributing any therapeutic benefits of a treatment. For instance, suppose we want to investigate the effectiveness of vitamin C in treating the common cold. We want to control for things such as how severe the participants' colds are. If we don't do that, the trial arm that receives vitamin C might suffer from less severe colds while the arm that receives the placebo suffers from worse colds. When we see that the placebo group took longer to recover, we would erroneously conclude that vitamin C is beneficial in treating the common cold.

The problem, Worrall argues, is that there are countlessly many possible confounding factors that we need to control for in order to ensure that the results of our RCTs are actually meaningful. And it is impossible to control for all of them. The best that researchers can do is to control for factors that they suspect *might* confound, and these decisions are based on background information. For instance, they might not control for the colors of the participants' shirts since we don't believe that one's garment color should affect one's response to vitamin C. The background information that researchers use include metaphysical narratives, and they tell us what the plausible and implausible confounding factors are.

As we saw, the acceptance of certain narratives is less epistemically justified than the orthodoxy would like us to believe. The result is that RCTs lead to a kind of deck-stacking: they can advance certain conclusions because the conclusions are consistent with our metaphysical narrative. In other words, when we get statistically significant results after we have controlled for all relevant factors, we conclude that the experimental treatment must be working. Our metaphysical narrative blinds us to the possibility of unknown confounding factors that we dismiss as implausible. As a result, we falsely believe that our RCT has demonstrated the efficacy of the treatment when in fact it could have been due to an implausible confounder. It is, in some respects, a feedback loop where experimental results are accepted because our metaphysical narrative tells us that we have controlled for all plausible confounders and the results of the experiment in turn further confirm the legitimacy of the narrative.

None of this is to say that RCTs are useless. But to think that they unproblematically provide the best of all types of evidence is to place faith in RCTs when arguments are wanting. At the very least, we should be aware of the philosophical challenges that one must overcome to elevate RCTs to the top of the evidential pecking order.

3.8 *P*-Hacking and Why Scientists Are Not All Bad People

In addition to the epistemic problems that we discussed earlier, there are challenging practical problems in the production of medical knowledge that are worth exploring. Although these problems might not appear to be philosophical at first, a realization that they are not isolated problems—but are consequences of sociopolitical institutions—might lead us to treat them systemically. To solve some of these problems, we will likely need to ask some basic questions of political philosophy: what is the purpose of the state? How do we balance individual liberty with collective desiderata?

One of the most illustrative examples of research challenges is the recent discussion of the *p*-hacking phenomenon. Since its introduction almost a century ago, *p*-value has become an important indicator for the significance of a research study. Its practical implications are vast: *p*-value dictates the acceptance of submissions for publications which in turns affects a researcher's professional trajectory, tenure-decision, funding, and so on.

In a nutshell, *p*-value measures the odds that a set of experimental results came about via pure chance. When we collect data, whatever statistical correlation that might exist between our variables can either be significant (e.g., reveal some nomological connection) or a matter of coincidence. We define the concept of a null-hypothesis as the claim that there is no (nomological) connection in the variable measured. A *p*-value of 0.05, for instance, tells us the probability that the observed results came about if the null-hypothesis is true is 5%. In other words, the probability that the results are mere coincidences is 5%.

The choice of 5% as the threshold for statistical significance is arbitrary. Indeed, in light of the Replication Crisis, a number of scholars have advocated the lowering *p*-value to 0.005 (or 0.5% for statistical significance) to ensure that only *really* significant results are considered well-established. With a higher statistical standard, we are more likely to replicate the results (at least of more rigorous studies). Nevertheless, if we adopt this standard, the results of much of our current scientific research would not be significant. One reason is that it would simply be too cumbersome and costly to run experiments that have a 0.005 *p*-value; they would require larger samples, longer duration, etc. Proponents of the change have suggested that we may need to relabel results that are currently "statistically significant" to "statistically suggestive" so that scientific research would not grind to a halt (Benjamin et al., 2018).

In the area of medical research, the translation of statistically significant results into bedside application is not a straightforward matter of choosing treatments that meet the *p*-value threshold. For starters, satisfying a *p*-value requirement does not actually tell us that we should accept the hypothesis being tested as true. For instance, suppose we know, prior to doing a study, that there is a remarkably slim chance (say, 1 in 20) that A is a beneficial treatment for condition X. Suppose after the study, we gather data that show there is a statistically significant correlation between receiving A and improved therapeutic outcomes. A study with a *p*-value of 0.05 would raise our confidence in the therapeutic benefits of A from 5% (our prior confidence) to 11%.[8] A study that meets the proper *p*-value requirement increases our confidence in A but it does not tell us whether our confidence in A is high enough to warrant our acceptance of it as a treatment. It all depends on the probability that A is therapeutically beneficial prior to our study. It might be the case that the study "nudges" the probability of A's effectiveness across the threshold of acceptable treatments. But by itself, *p*-value does not tell us *where* that threshold is, or whether the treatment has met that threshold.

From the point of view of clinical reasoning, *p*-value is but one of a host of considerations when translating research results into clinical recommendations. There are uncertainties in even the most trusted treatments, and our willingness to tolerate the risks depends on a treatment's potential benefits and the availability of other more promising alternatives. We might, for instance, be willing to tolerate greater risks because a treatment in question presents the only viable response to a debilitating disease. The fact that a treatment has a moderate risk of being therapeutically useless might be overlooked, if the choice of no treatment leads to terrible outcomes.

Given the emphasis on *p*-value in research and funding, there is a strong incentive to engage only in clinical research that would lead to results that satisfy the 0.05 magic number. Suppose the only way to study certain treatment options is to conduct trials that could *not* satisfy the 0.05 standard (perhaps getting enough subjects would simply be too costly). The practical pressure to produce results that meet the 0.05 threshold would thus create a disincentive to conduct these statistically less significant trials. By singularly conducting studies that have 0.05 *p*-value, we could actually decrease the therapeutic options that are available before us. Clinicians and patients will not have the opportunity to consider less certain treatments simply because fewer have been studied. In situations where less certain treatments are better than none, the quality of clinical care would actually decrease in light of a rigid adherence to 0.05.

It is widely known that researchers can manipulate experimental data in order to generate statistically significant results. Some of these practices are clearly unethical.[9] While the practice of pharmaceutical companies paying prominent researchers to sign their names to studies that the researchers played no part in ("ghost writing") raises issues of conflicts of interests and scientific objectivity, the use of "ghost management"—manipulations by pharmaceutical companies to control research, writing, and publication of results—is more disconcerting (Sismondo, 2007). It involves wholesale control of the dissemination of information by gaming the publication process.[10] These are transparently problematic cases that potentially add biased studies and results into our corpus of accepted scientific beliefs. Regardless of their frequency (Sismondo argues that they are disturbingly common), bad science undercuts the trust we have in medical knowledge and the trust the public has in our fidelity.

Although blatant attempts to massage data like the ones mentioned are certainly unacceptable, *p*-hackings often involve far less nefarious actors and questionable motives. Indeed, the ubiquitous nature of *p*-hacking is partly the result of researchers following the letters of the research laws (but, perhaps, not the spirit). In their 2015 paper, Megan Head et al. conclude that not only is *p*-hacking widespread, researchers often do not even consider some of their research practices as illegitimate collections of experimental data. Head et al. identify some common ways researchers can game the data in order to obtain a 0.05 *p*-value. They include:

- Conducting statistical analyses midway through experiments to decide whether to continue collecting data;
- Recording many response variables and deciding which to report post-analysis;
- Deciding whether to include or drop outliers post-analysis;
- Excluding, combining, or splitting treatment groups post-analysis;
- Including or excluding covariates post-analysis; and
- Stopping data exploration if an analysis yields a significant *p*-value (Head, Holman, Lanfear, Kahn, & Jennions, 2015, para. 2).

In a 2002 article, Leslie John, et al. (cited in Head et al., 2015) surveyed 2,000 psychiatrists to determine how often they engage in *p*-hacking. Respondents were asked to rate whether they thought their practices were defensible using 0 for no, 1 for maybe, and 2 for yes. For the item "Deciding whether to collect more data after looking to see whether the results were significant," over 50% of the psychiatrists surveyed admitted anonymously to the practice and rated it above a mean of 1.5, meaning a large number of researchers were letting the 0.05 statistical goal guide their research, and that many of them did not see this as problematic. Unlike the more egregious examples before, these subtler forms of data manipulations are often not conscious or deliberate acts of academic fraud.

A number of academics have suggested ways we can combat or minimize the risks of *p*-hacking. From requiring researchers to disclose all raw data to mandating that the length of data collection be fixed before the trials begin, from blindly conducting data analyses to explicitly stating one's statistical methodologies, the

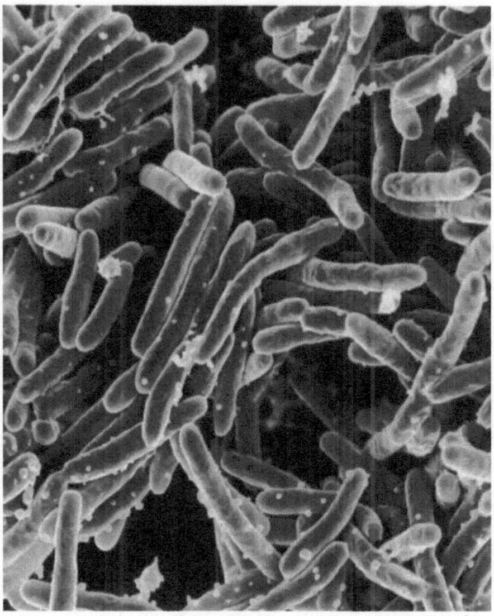

FIGURE 3.3 Electron Micrograph of *Mycobacterium tuberculosis*

About 10 million people globally contract TB annually and about 1.7 million people die from it. The U.S. provided $264 million through USAID in FY 2018 to help fight the disease. The amount is budgeted to decrease by $63 million in 2019. The emergence of antibiotic-resistant TB poses a grave global health threat. *Source:* Image from www.flickr.com/photos/niaid/5149398678/.

responses have largely focused on educating researchers on how to become better scientists. Nevertheless, as we look at practical changes that can improve research, we ought to look at the broader issues that confront researchers *qua* social beings. The fact of the matter is that researchers work within a fairly regimented system, with incentives and disincentives set up to steer particular types of research and outcomes. One of the more significant revelations of the Replication Crisis is that results from well-known experiments are rarely replicated. A cornerstone of peer review is that one must present one's research results in such a manner that fellow researchers can confirm the discoveries. Nevertheless, in an intellectual market where young academics seldom gain tenure by replicating other researchers' experiments, there is a perverse incentive not to play the role of scorekeeper. Just as the appetite of baseball fans to see homeruns encourages hitters to be sluggers, when the market sets certain preferences, researchers are likely to follow the incentives. To do otherwise is to engage in a kind of intellectual martyrdom: it is supererogatory when there are bills to be paid.

Academic publishing, university funding, and the dissemination of scientific knowledge all adopt certain sub-optimal and occasionally epistemically self-defeating knowledge production systems because of the presence of perverse incentives. Consider a savvy layperson who appreciates scientific discoveries but has little access to academic journals. She is likely going to receive her scientific news from popular media. A headline that screams "Scientists Identify the Breast Cancer Gene" will likely garner more clicks and more reads than one that says "Scientists Continue to Confirm the Benefits of Standard Treatments." News outlets have every incentive to disseminate information that generates revenue. As important as it is to be honest, objective, and responsible in the age of hyper-competitive media, profit is clearly a consideration of how and what to publish.

Similarly, universities are more likely to receive grant money for groundbreaking research projects than replications of known results. Then Vice President Joe Biden asked for an initiative to find a cure for cancer in 2016. Congress promptly allocated $1.8 billion to the effort over seven years. In terms of well-confirmed evidence, we know that diet and exercise can significantly affect our health outcomes; yet, the public craves silver bullets. The same pressure that compels doctors to write unnecessary prescriptions for antsy patients is the same pressure that pushes researchers towards finding a physiochemical cure.

The sensational nature of scientific news often distorts our research priorities. Ebola became a media hot button topic in 2014, and the U.S. Congress quickly allocated $5.2 billion to an emergency bill to combat the disease. Yet, in 2015, Ebola killed about 11,000 people worldwide while antibiotic-resistant infections killed over 700,000 people during the same year. Congress allocated only $1.2 billion to confront the latter—a unquestionably deadlier long-term public health threat (The Data Team, 2015). Politicians respond to their constituents' concerns and these concerns might not necessarily align with responsible research. Like media outlets, politicians are merely doing their jobs, and the combinations of these agents all doing what they believe are their professional responsibilities creates a system of knowledge production such that *p*-hacking and other less than ideal research practices emerge. To single out scientists as the sole causes of flawed research is to miss the systemic problems. It asks scientists alone to bear the cost of a better system of knowledge production. Not only would this be unfair, its chances of success are slim. After all, so long as there are incentives to meeting a particular benchmark, researchers will continue (consciously or otherwise) to work to meet those benchmarks.

One of the insights of Kuhn's work on the philosophy of science is his recognition of the importance of the social components of scientific research. Scientists are social beings affected by psychological biases, communal pressures, and financial incentives. As long as we are interested in understanding how *we* do science (not as some abstract rational experimental machines), we must understand how these forces affect the production of knowledge. Like all creatures susceptible to conditioning, we do what we are incentivized to do. Without the proverbial cheese at the end of the maze, we just sit at the starting line. At the same time, if the incentives do not align with the goals of knowledge production, we will forever be led astray. The question is whether we can create a system of knowledge production within a free market system that can be incentivized to do what is best for us. It might turn out to be the case that we cannot have our cake and eat it too.

Notes

1 For an overview and the scope of the crisis, see Baker (2016). An article by The Open Science Collaboration (2015) on the difficulties of replicating results from psychological sciences is widely credited for sparking the current movement. For a provocative discussion of the issue in oncology, see Begley and Ellis (2012).

2 Over the course of a week, I chatted with Adelina multiple times. Although my encounter with her could have been an elaborate ruse to trick a young college student, I certainly left with the impression that Adelina was sincere.

3 See Chapter 3 of Goodman (1983).

4 To appreciate the evidential symmetry between green and grue, for every instance of an emerald that is green, we also find an emerald that is grue. Thus, "All emeralds are green" has as many positive instances as "All emeralds are grue" and vice versa.

5 The idea that a cause can lead to an effect in the past is often referred to as "backward causation." Many philosophers, including Immanuel Kant, consider backward causation impossible. Kant, for instance, considered the claim "effects precede their causes" a conceptual truth. However, research in quantum mechanics raises at least the physical possibility of backward causation. Wheeler-Feynman absorber theory, for instance, interprets quantum electrodynamics in a temporally invariant manner. The theory offers the most elegant and plausible solutions to electromagnetic fields equations, but it violates the classical notion that causes must precede effects. In other words, it permits the possibility of backward causation.

6 According to pessimistic induction, the fact that most, if not all, of our past theories have been false is evidence that our current theories are very likely false. Of course, plenty of the theories we current hold make accurate predictions. The combination of these two claims means that making true predictions may have little to do with a theory being true.

7 There is a connection between our discussion here and the earlier discussion regarding the aim of medicine. If medicine merely looks to improve our lots and not to discover and learn about the nature of our physiology, then these issues would become less pressing. As soon as medicine claims to be an epistemic activity—a pursuit of truth—then medicine must address the gap between what works and what is true.

8 For a terrific overview of the limitations and misunderstandings of *p*-value, see Nuzzo (2014).

9 It is obviously difficult to determine the extent to which deliberate data fraud exists in scientific research. George and Buyse (2015) conclude that there is no reliable evidence to indicate that data fraud is common. However, well publicized cases often undermine trust in medical research, and George and Buyse recommend a cost-effective way to monitor data collection and use.

10 Evidence that clinical trials sponsored by pharmaceutical companies favor the companies' products is widely available and well-substantiated. For example, see Lexchin, Bero, Djulbegovic, and Clark (2003).

References

Baker, M. (2016). 1,500 scientists lift the lid on reproducibility. *Nature, 533*(7604), 452–454.

Begley, C. G., & Ellis, L. M. (2012). Raise standards for preclinical cancer research. *Nature, 483*, 531. doi:10.1038/483531a

Benjamin, D. J., Berger, J. O., Johannesson, M., Nosek, B. A., Wagenmakers, E. J., Berk, R., . . . Johnson, V. E. (2018). Redefine statistical significance. *Nature Human Behaviour, 2*(1), 6–10. doi:10.1038/s41562-017-0189-z

George, S. L., & Buyse, M. (2015). Data fraud in clinical trials. *Clinical Investigation, 5*(2), 161–173. doi:10.4155/cli.14.116

Goodman, N. (1983). *Fact, fiction, and forecast* (4th ed.). Cambridge, MA: Harvard University Press.

Guyatt, G., Cairns, J., Churchill, D., et al. (1992). Evidence-based medicine: A new approach to teaching the practice of medicine. *JAMA, 268*(17), 2420–2425. doi:10.1001/jama.1992.03490170092032

Harbour, R., & Miller, J. (2001). A new system for grading recommendations in evidence based guidelines. *BMJ: British Medical Journal, 323*(7308), 334–336.

Head, M. L., Holman, L., Lanfear, R., Kahn, A. T., & Jennions, M. D. (2015). The extent and consequences of p-hacking in science. *PLOS Biology, 13*(3), e1002106. doi:10.1371/journal.pbio.1002106

John, L. K., Loewenstein, G., & Prelec, D. (2012). Measuring the prevalence of questionable research practices with incentives for truth telling. *Psychological Science, 23*(5), 524–532. doi:10.1177/0956797611430953

Leibovici, L. (2001). Effects of remote, retroactive intercessory prayer on outcomes in patients with bloodstream infection: Randomised controlled trial. *BMJ: British Medical Journal, 323*(7327), 1450–1451.

Lexchin, J., Bero, L. A., Djulbegovic, B., & Clark, O. (2003). Pharmaceutical industry sponsorship and research outcome and quality: Systematic review. *BMJ: British Medical Journal, 326*(7400), 1167–1167.

Nuzzo, R. (2014, February 13). *Scientific method: Statistical errors. Nature,* 506, 150–152. doi:10.1038/506150a

Rosen, G. (2010). Metaphysical dependence: Grounding and reduction. In B. Hale & A. Hoffmann (Eds.), *Modality: Metaphysics, logic, and epistemology* (pp. 109–136). New York, NY: Oxford University Press.

Schorge, J. O., McCann, C., & Del Carmen, M. G. (2010). Surgical debulking of ovarian cancer: What difference does it make? *Reviews in Obstetrics and Gynecology, 3*(3), 111–117.

Sismondo, S. (2007). Ghost management: How much of the medical literature is shaped behind the scenes by the pharmaceutical industry? *PLOS Medicine, 4*(9), e286. doi:10.1371/journal.pmed.0040286

The Data Team. (2015, May 10). The toll of a tragedy. *The Economist.*

The Open Science Collaboration. (2015). Estimating the reproducibility of psychological science. *Science, 349*(6251).

Worrall, J. (2007). Evidence in medicine and evidence-based medicine. *Philosophy Compass, 2*(6), 981–1022.

4

EXPLANATIONS IN MEDICINE

4.1 Do We Need Explanations in the Sciences?

We all know that the sky is blue, but fewer of us can say *why* it is so. Explanations intuitively provide more information than knowledge alone. Indeed, it seems that in order to practice medicine (and even science in general), we often don't need to know why something happens. For instance, a number of studies have shown that frequent consumption of hot liquids such as green tea leads to increased risk of gastric cancer (e.g., see Mao et al., 2011). So, a physician might recommend to someone who is concerned about gastric cancer that she should avoid hot tea, even though researchers don't quite know *why* consuming hot liquids leads to increased risks. Similarly, electroconvulsive therapy is an effective short-term treatment for depression. In fact, some studies, including one from The UK ECT Review Group (2003), show that it outperforms drug therapies. But researchers have limited knowledge of *why* sending electricity through the brains of patients with depression can improve their conditions. If all we care about is improving health outcomes of patients, then the search for answers to the "why" questions seems to be an epistemic cherry on top.[1]

To be sure, there is something deeply satisfying knowing why things behave the way the they do. For instance, Newton's laws of motion, along with his universal law of gravitation, explain all three of Kepler's laws:

(1) Planets move in elliptical orbits;
(2) For a given duration, the orbits of a planet mark equal areas around the sun; and
(3) The square of a period in the revolution a planet is proportional to the cube of the semi-major axis of the orbit.

Newton's theory not only allows us to logically derive Kepler's laws in the sense that they are merely narrower instances of Newton's more general laws; it also

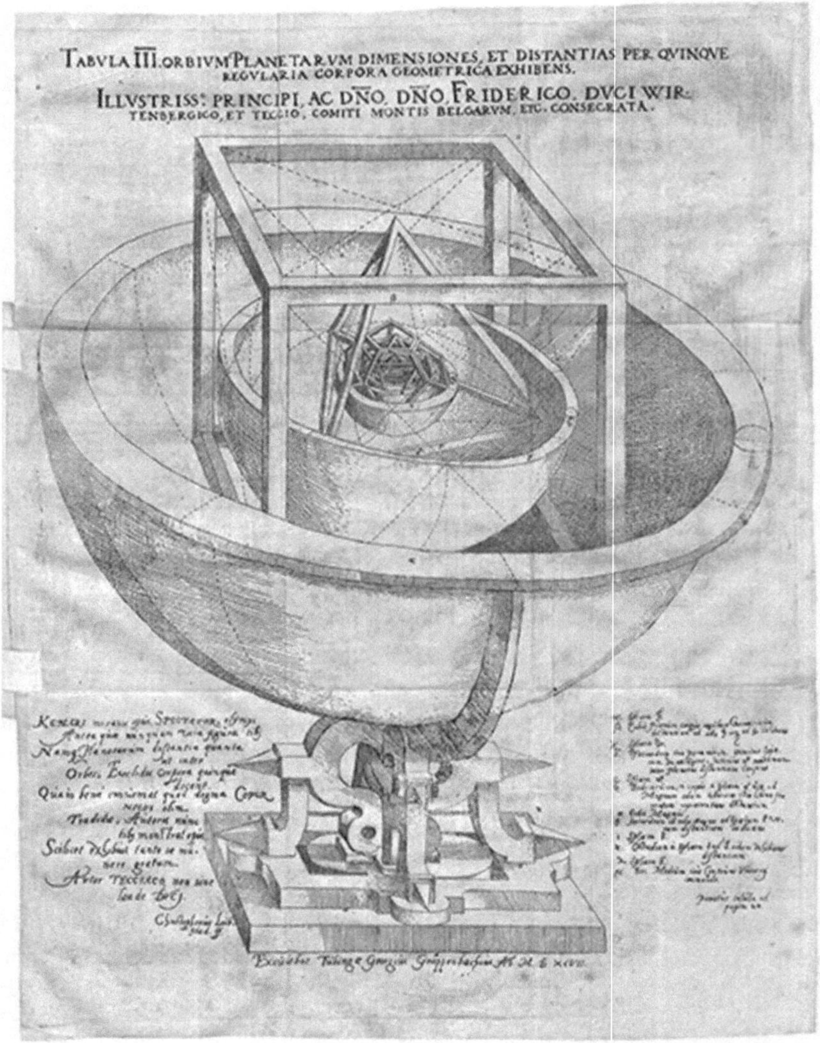

FIGURE 4.1 Kepler's Solar System

In his earlier work *Mysterium Cosmographium* (*The Secret of the Universe*), published in 1596—a full 13 years before the publication of his legendary three laws—Kepler suggested that the orbits of the planets mark out areas between the planetary spheres and that they conform to nesting Platonic solids.

explains why Kepler's laws are true. As planets travel closer to the sun, they accelerate in accordance with Newton's theory of gravity, and, as they slingshot away, they decelerate. And this result explains Kepler's second law. If one were interested in no more than predicting the location of a planet on any given night, Kepler's laws might suffice. What Newton shows is that Kepler's laws are in fact specific instances of more fundamental physical laws. In reducing Kepler's laws to his laws, Newton goes beyond refining Kepler's discovery; he provides an explanation for Kepler's laws (and planetary motion in general).

The search for explanations seems to be the penultimate goal of scientific endeavors. We don't just want to know what is the case; we also want to know why it is the case. In fact, Newton was unsatisfied with his account of gravity and mass. Fearing that attributing an intrinsic power of gravitational attraction to mass strayed dangerously close to the Scholastics' practice of introducing some hidden power whenever an explanation is wanting, Newton suggested that the day would come when we can explain why mass attracts. It was arguably not until Einstein's thesis more than 200 years later that explained how gravity is curvature in space-time that we get the semblance of an explanation.[2]

Within the field of philosophy of science, there is a heated debate as to whether science should be troubled with the search for explanations. Philosophers such as Bas van Fraassen see explanations as adding nothing more to empirical research than what mere descriptions of the observable can already do (van Fraassen, 1980, especially chapter 5). Explanations, they argue, provide only psychological comfort—a sort of story-telling that eases our instinctive desire to understand. These stories might be true or false. But if we can make successful predictions, and if we can account for all the empirical observations (van Fraassen calls it empirical adequacy), we can remain entirely agnostic with regards to whether the stories we tell are true.

Banishing explanations to the realm of psychological story-telling is particularly disconcerting when we notice the assumed relationship between a hypothesis' ability to explain and its truth. Often referred to as "inference to the best explanation" (IBE) or "abductive reasoning" (a term coined by the American Pragmatist Charles Sanders Peirce), countless everyday practices involve inferring the truth of a hypothesis on the basis of its explanatory power. A police investigator examines tire tracks, the location of the vehicles, and the dents on the cars, and she infers that a vehicle ran a stop sign and was hit by another one at the intersection. She thinks the hypothesis is plausible because it best explains the observation. If explanations are nothing but story-telling, then inference to the best explanation would be in trouble; what gives us psychological comfort need not be true after all. The stakes cannot be higher: if philosophers like van Fraassen are right, the search for explanations is not only unnecessary for the practice of science, they are nothing but quests to make us sleep better at night. Why bother with explanations when you can just take an Ambien?

On the other hand, philosophers like Hilary Putnam have argued that explanations are a valuable part of science. Without understanding why things happen the way that they do, our successes in science are reduced to miracles (Putnam, 1975). If we have no explanation for why sugar dissolves in water, the fact that a cube of sugar dissolves in our next cup of tea would be yet another instance in a long chain of lucky outcomes. The (regularly observed) solubility of sugar would literally be inexplicable. To justify confidence in our predictions (that the sugar cube *will* dissolve when placed in water), we need to find the underlying nomological connections that are responsible for sugar's solubility. These nomological connections are, of course, not directly observable; we must infer them. The most common way to do so is to use IBE. Explanations become a critical tool not only for making sense of the world, but also for helping us learn about parts of the universe that are unobservable by direct human perception.

4.2 The Stories of Semmelweis and Goldberger: How Explanations Saved Lives

In 1851, Hungarian obstetrician Ignaz Semmelweis noticed something distressing in his obstetric clinic in Vienna General Hospital—a leading hospital in Europe and a center of medical education. Pregnant women who gave birth at the clinic had an alarmingly higher rate of "childbed fever" than those who gave births at home, or even en route to the hospital. The difference, some have estimated, was anywhere from 10 to 20 times higher. Childbed fever was a particularly dangerous risk of childbirth: as many as one in three women would die from it. Symptoms include persistent high fever, excruciating abdominal pain, organ failure, stroke, and septic shock.

Semmelweis considered a host of possible explanations for the elevated instances of childbed fever at his hospital. He thought, for instance, that the sight of priests walking by the maternity ward to deliver last rites might be depressing women enough to cause the deadly fever. To test the hypothesis, he had the priests walk a different route. The measure, however, proved futile. He also hypothesized that the position of delivery might be the cause and he instituted an entirely different birthing position. The effort was again to no avail.[3]

One fateful day, a medical student injured a colleague of Semmelweis with a scalpel during an autopsy. The colleague developed symptoms strikingly similar to those of childbed fever. Semmelweis theorized that the man must have been exposed to cadaveric material— "morbid poison." It was this unobservable poison, Semmelweis suggested, that caused childbed fever to spike in his hospital. He proposed a rigorous regiment of handwashing with chlorinated lime solution. The rate of childbed fever plummeted.[4] Years later, scientists would learn that the morbid poison was none other than Group A *hemolytic Streptococcus* bacteria. Obviously, Semmelweis could not observe the bacteria. In fact, his understanding of the vector of "childbed fever" was limited to some unobservable morbid poison whose detection was done largely by smell. Still, by using IBE, Semmelweis inferred the existence of microscopic entities that were responsible for the infections, and he further confirmed his hypothesis by correctly predicting that antiseptic wash would decrease their transmission.[5]

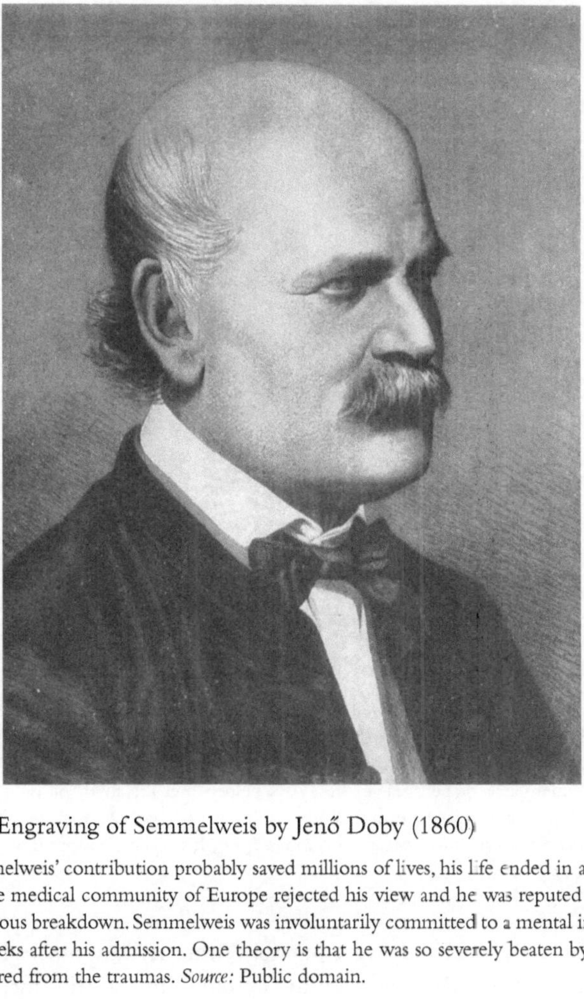

FIGURE 4.2 Engraving of Semmelweis by Jenő Doby (1860)

Although Semmelweis' contribution probably saved millions of lives, his life ended in a less than dignified fashion. The medical community of Europe rejected his view and he was reputed to have suffered episodes of nervous breakdown. Semmelweis was involuntarily committed to a mental institution where he died two weeks after his admission. One theory is that he was so severely beaten by the guards that he never recovered from the traumas. *Source:* Public domain.

Medical breakthroughs like Semmelweis' pepper the history of medicine. In 1914, the U.S. Surgeon General Rupert Blue asked the renowned American epidemiologist Joseph Goldberger to investigate the high rate of pellagra in the American South. Pellagra is a potentially fatal condition characterized by the four Ds: diarrhea, dermatitis, dementia, and death. Goldberger noticed that pellagra affected mostly the poor, such as sharecroppers. More puzzlingly, staff in hospitals who took care of patients with pellagra rarely developed it. The demographic patterns of pellagra patients simply did not match the conventional wisdom at the time, which assumed that pellagra was spread by germs. Goldberger conducted a series of experiments in orphanages and prisons to test his hypothesis that pellagra was not an infectious disease, but rather stemmed from poor diet. In the Rankin Farm experiment, Goldberger asked 11 prisoners to switch to a rudimentary diet

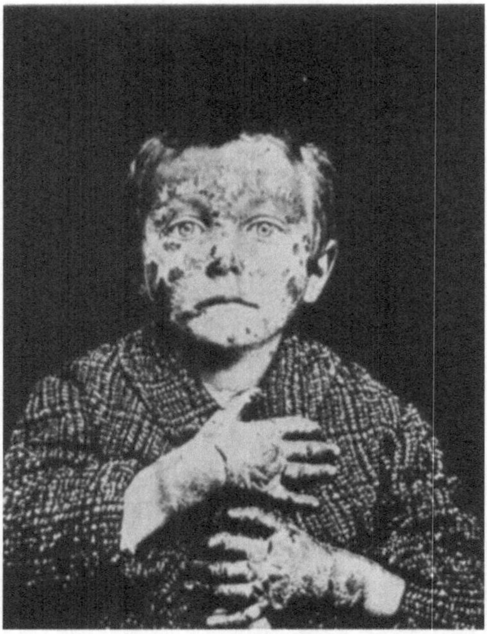

FIGURE 4.3 A European Young Boy with Pellagra around 1910s

Pellagra was widespread in Europe as well, primarily in Northern Italy and Northern Spain where a corn-heavy diet introduced from the New World was common. "Pellagra" literally means "sour skin" in Italian. Since individuals with pellagra were sensitive to sunlight, some scholars have suggested that the emergence of pellagra in the 1700s helped fuel the myth of vampires. See Hampl and Hampl (1997). *Source:* Image from: Casimir Funk's 1914 book *Die Vitamine; ihre Bedeutung fur die Physiologie und Pathologie mit vesonderer Berucksichtigung*, https://collections.nlm.nih.gov/catalog/nlm:nlmuid-101434598-img.

of grits, biscuits, cabbage, and sweet potato. Within five months, all 11 prisoners had developed pellagra. But the scientific community was still unconvinced that pellagra was the result of diet and not caused by infectious agents. In a dramatic demonstration, Goldberger injected himself, his wife, and 14 other volunteers with the blood drawn from pellagra patients. None of them developed the disease.[6,7] It was not for another 20 years that researchers discovered pellagra was the result of B vitamin niacin deficiency. In 1940, the Committee on Food and Nutrition (known as the Food and Nutrition Board now) recommended fortifying flour with niacin (along with iron, thiamin, and riboflavin), and diet-based cases of pellagra dropped from approximately 230,000 cases per year in 1928 to virtual elimination in the United States today (Clay, Schmick, Troesken, & National Bureau of Economic Research, 2017).

In both Semmelweis' and Goldberger's case, the use of inference to the best explanation allows them to infer the most plausible hypotheses that best explain the evidence. The rough logical structure of IBE is as follows:

TABLE 4.1 The relationship between hypotheses and observation

Hypothesis (e.g., pellagra is caused by poor diets)

Hypothesis' ability to explain the observation.

Observations (e.g., mostly poor people develop pellagra, the rate of pellagra drops when there is a switch to a more balanced diet, injecting oneself with the blood of a pellagra patient does not induce pellagra, etc.)

One of the important characteristics of IBE is that the conclusions always contain elements of things or events that are unobserved. Both Semmelweis and Goldberger could not observe the causal agents of their respective pathologies. In case of Goldberger, the most he could articulate was that the cause of pellagra had something to do with the patients' diets.

Although some philosophers object to the use of IBE even in the most pedestrian cases involving unobserved hypothesis (e.g., reconstructing car crashes from observations gathered at the accident scenes), the real point of contention with IBE has been its use to infer the existence of unobservables. By definition, unobservables are those entities that we *cannot* observe unaided. Some of the traditional examples include electrons, germs, viruses, genes, gravity, other people's subjective mental experiences, and metaphysical connections such as causality and nomological necessitation. In 1801, British scientist Thomas Young conducted his ingenious double-slit experiment. He was shocked to see that light did not travel through the slits and create two bright lines on the screen; instead, the slits cast a series of blurry vertical lines of varying intensity. If light consisted of streams of particles, as proponents of the corpuscular theory (including Newton) believed, one would expect two lines. Young concluded that light was in fact not made of particles, but of waves.

Young's wave conclusion was not directly observed; it was rather the result of deploying IBE. He inferred the wave-like nature of light because the wave hypothesis best explained the absence of two clear vertical lines and the varying intensities of the series of illuminated spots. Unlike reconstructing a car crash, Young's experiment involved inferences of not just something (i.e., light as wave) that he did not observe; it involved something he *could* not observe unaided. The world around us contains things that we can observe with our sensory organs and it contains things that we cannot observe. Inference to the best explanations promises to give us the logical tools to "see" into the unobservable parts of the

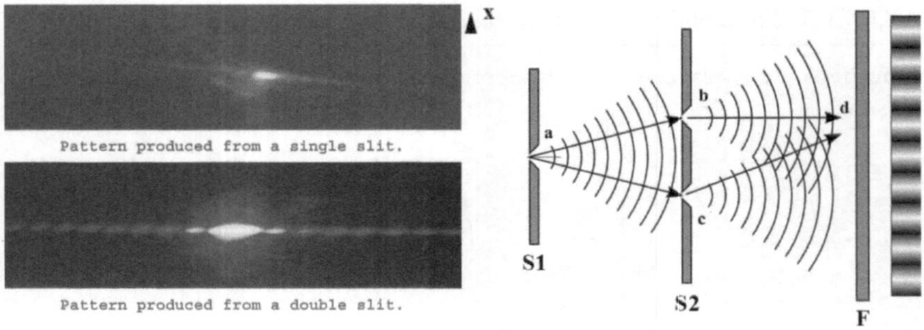

FIGURE 4.4 Double-Slit Experiment

Source: Image on the left created by Patrick Edwin Moran and can be found at https://commons.wikimedia.org/wiki/File:Single_%26_double_slit_experiment.jpg. Image on the right created by Wikipedia user Lacatosias and can be found at https://commons.wikimedia.org/wiki/File:Ebohr1.png.

world. Without IBE, it is difficult to fathom how we can learn about the parts of the universe that lie beyond the narrow limits of our perceptions. To reject IBE amounts to closing the scientific door to discovering vast portions of the universe.

4.3 Elegance and Useful Falsehoods: The Limits of IBE

Given how familiar and important IBE is to how we theorize about the world, why would anyone think that it is problematic? Many philosophers, especially empiricists (those who believe knowledge can only be derived from sense experience), have rejected the legitimacy of IBE for a host of reasons. We will consider three of the more challenging objections to IBE.

The "best of the bad lot" objection points to the fact that IBE claims that we ought to accept a hypothesis because it is the best explanation for the evidence. But "best" is a comparative evaluation. Suppose a loud banging noise is coming from under my car hood. I wonder what's causing the noise and my fellow passenger responds, "I know exactly what it is. It is a gremlin banging against the inside of your hood!" Suppose I reject his "hypothesis" because I think it's absurd. He adds, "Well, here is another hypothesis. It is not a gremlin, but that there is a family of gremlins living under the hood and one of them is banging about." Now, if you think it is ridiculous that his initial hypothesis explains the noise, this second hypothesis is even more ridiculous. So, according to inference to the best explanation, you ought to accept the first hypothesis. Obviously, this is a bad use of IBE, but exactly what is the defect? This "best of a bad lot" objection will resurface when we examine Kathleen Okruhlik's views on the role of values in scientific inquiries in the final chapter.

A second problem with IBE exploits the underdeterminacy of non-deductive reasoning. A finite amount of evidence can never single out one explanation as the only explanation. As such, we must ask which one of a host of explanations is

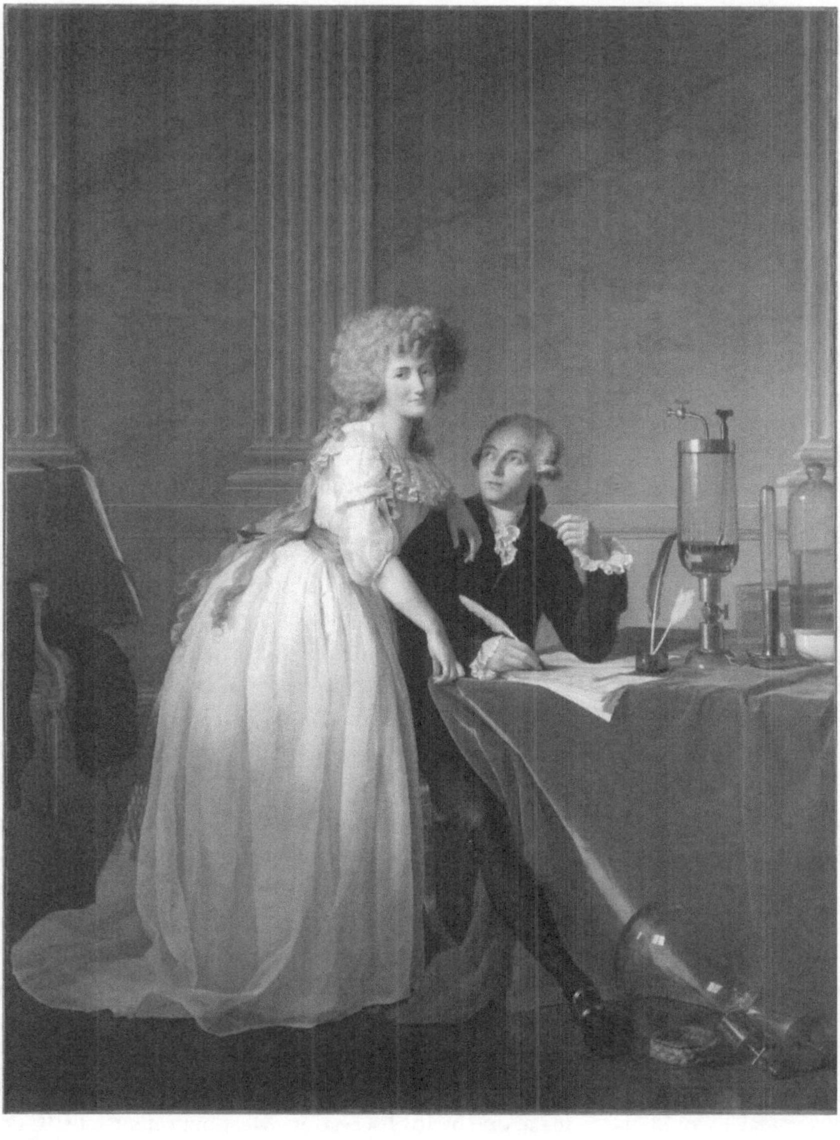

FIGURE 4.5 Portrait of Lavoisier

Jacques Louis David's 1788 painting of the French chemist Antoine Laurent Lavoisier and his brilliant wife Marie Anne Pierrette Paulze, who assisted him in his research. Lavoisier cast serious doubts on the phlogiston theory of combustion when his experiments in the 1780s showed that the heating of some metals led to their increase in weight. According to the phlogiston theory, as metals are heated, phlogistons would escape and the metal would lose weight. Many proponents held onto the phlogiston theory, and some even proposed that phlogiston has a negative weight, which explained Lavoisier's observations. Lavoisier went on to discover oxygen (from the Greek for "acid generator") because he (erroneously) believed that all acids contain oxygen. Unrelatedly, Lavoisier was guillotined during the chaos of the French Revolution. The court, however, admitted a year and a half after his execution that he was falsely convicted, much to his hypothetical chagrin. *Source:* Public domain.

the best. Consider again the car noise example. Suppose there are two hypotheses. H_1 says that I had likely forgotten to tighten a belt in the engine after working on it earlier in the day and the belt is now flopping against the inside of the hood, making a banging noise. H_2, on the other hand, says exactly the same, except there is a gremlin as well. Obviously, commonsense dictates that we ought to reject H_2. For one thing, the addition of the gremlin does no extra explanatory work; it is merely an epicycle spinning by itself unconnected to any part of the explanation. Yet, our preference for H_1 seems to rely on some notion of simplicity or explanatory elegance. These concepts, however intuitive they appear, require explications and justifications, especially when we use them to infer the plausibility of a hypothesis. Why should we believe that the simplest hypothesis is in fact the most plausible? What do we mean by "simple" anyway?

Finally, the history of science has shown us that false theories can be extremely good at providing plausible explanations. Young's hypothesis that light consists of waves seemingly offered a great explanation for what he observed. We now know that light is not a wave but exhibits a wave-particle duality. Likewise, the phlogiston theory of combustion championed by European chemists in the 18th century suggests that during combustion, phlogiston (a substance that is fire-based) is released from metal leaving behind oxide. The theory nicely explains calcination (a heating process by which metals decompose) and the oxidation that occasionally follows. Moreover, it also explains why heating oxide (or calx, as it was known then) in charcoal powder can result in new metal; phlogiston theorists claimed that charcoal was rich in phlogiston and that the heating process reintroduced phlogiston back into the oxide. As we now know, phlogiston does not exist; yet, as a dominant theory in chemistry, it did a wonderful job of explaining various experimental observations. In fact, phlogiston theory is not even approximately true since it posits a substance that has no counterpart in reality at all (unlike, say, Semmelweis' morbid poison which was later identified as bacteria). The history of science is littered with false theories that were often accepted on the basis of their alleged explanatory power. The connection that IBE defenders wish to establish between the explanatory power of a hypothesis and its truth seems to fly in the face of the history of science.

These objections cannot be easily dismissed. Rather than addressing them piecemeal, I would like to make one basic observation. Most opponents of IBE do not reject its use in cases for drawing conclusions that contain only observables. My friend borrows my bicycle and when he returns it, I see fine grains of sand embedded in the tire treads. I conclude that my friend rode it to the nearby beach. When I see him later in the evening, I ask if he had done so and he replies that he did. I infer from the evidence and his answer that he in fact did ride to the beach. Could he have lied? Of course! But it is far more likely that he was being truthful.

I was not there to observe his trek, but I use IBE to make the plausible inference. This sort of inference is so common that if we were to reject it, it would be exceedingly difficult to get through a normal day. Our legal system, for instance, relies on the legitimacy of IBE. We infer from the evidence and witnesses' testimonies the intentions of the defendant. Did he *intend* to harm the victim or was it an accident? Was he *aware* that there were alternative courses of action available? These are mental states that no one other than the defendant could observe.

The question before us is this: how come we have no fundamental problem relying on IBE to infer conclusions about events that are unobserved but observable, yet we reject them when they are unobservable? Recall that the definition of an unobservable is that which we cannot observe unaided. Why would the inferential legitimacy of IBE—a mode of logical reasoning—be dependent on our very contingent biological limitations? It is akin to concluding that the principle of addition only works for numbers we can keep in our heads but not for those that are too large to hold. If IBE "works" for inferring unobserved but observable conclusions, then it should also work for inferring conclusions that we cannot in principle observe.

Dinosaurs are observable in the sense that if they were parading in front of us right now, we *could* observe them without instruments. Bacteria, on the other hand, are not. But until we are able to clone dinosaurs and bring them back to existence, the only way to observe dinosaurs is to travel back in time to see them with our naked eyes. The chances of us seeing dinosaurs are on a par with our chances to observe a bacterium with our naked eyes: it is logically possible that in some fantastic sense we *could* modify our visual cortex to enable seeing into the world of bacteria. Yet, somehow most opponents of IBE maintain that we can legitimately use IBE to infer the existence of dinosaurs but not bacteria. The difference between unobservables and unobserved (but observable) cannot be merely the greater risk of making mistakes when we posit the former vs. the latter. Using IBE to infer the existence of dinosaurs exposes us to risks of being wrong that are not substantially different from inferring the existence of bacteria. To insist that somehow unobservables are in a worse position strikes me as arbitrary.

Nevertheless, the use of IBE as a main tool in theoretical reasoning is far from unproblematic. When researchers or clinicians infer the cause of a disease, our confidence in whether their theories are correct depend on the connection between plausibility and the explanatory power of the theories. The three objections we outlined raise serious doubts that the connection exists. Even if there is no fundamental difference between observables and unobservables with regard to the use of IBE, it could very well be the case that they are *both* in trouble. As long as we think medicine involves delivering true claims about our physiology, there is an implicit assumption that a tie exists between plausibility/truth and the explanatory power of a hypothesis. Randomized clinical trials, for instance, infer the plausibility of a hypothesis on the basis of the trial's observations. For example, subjects in the active arm improved and the subjects in the controlled arm did not; thus, the best hypothesis to explain the difference is that the therapy being tested is beneficial. Without a solid justification for IBE, both clinical and research medicine would rest on a shaky epistemic foundation.

4.4 Two Ways to Explain Explanations

To understand the logic of IBE, we obviously need to understand what an explanation is. Without a proper theory of explanation, we cannot tell whether a hypothesis actually explains the observations. Contemporary theories of explanations largely fall into two camps: explanations are either mind-independent or they are mind-dependent/epistemic.

A mind-independent theory of explanation says that whether A explains B consists of an objective relationship between the two. For instance, I might say that A explains B because A is the cause of B. And, if causation is an objective relationship, then whether A explains B is mind-independent in the sense that the explanation relation between the two exists regardless of whether anyone knows it, cares about it, understands it, etc.

One of the classic mind-independent theories of explanations is the deductive-nomological model offered by Austrian empiricist Carl Hempel (1905–1997). Hempel suggests that explanations are in fact logical arguments consisting of premises and conclusions. The premises of the argument do the explaining and the conclusion is the thing that is explained or is the object of the explanations. He calls the former "explanans" and the latter "explanandum." There are three basic requirements for an adequate explanation:

(1) The truth of premises guarantees the truth of the conclusion (the definition of validity);
(2) A law of nature plays an indispensable role in the inference (that is, the law cannot just be included among the premises and does no actual inferential work); and
(3) The premises are true.

Suppose I notice that the soap bubbles from my dishwashing expand on the countertop and I want to know why. A typical Hempelian explanation looks something like this:

(1) Air expands when heated.
(2) The soap bubbles that I made contained heated air (from the hot water).

Therefore, the soap bubbles expanded.

This is a valid argument in that if the premises are true, the conclusion must be true. And, premise (1) of the argument is a law of nature. So long as both the premises are true, the argument satisfies Hempel's definition of an adequate explanation for why the soap bubbles expanded.

Although Hempel's model is well-known among philosophers of science, its ingenuity is often underappreciated. When we explain in ordinary contexts, we

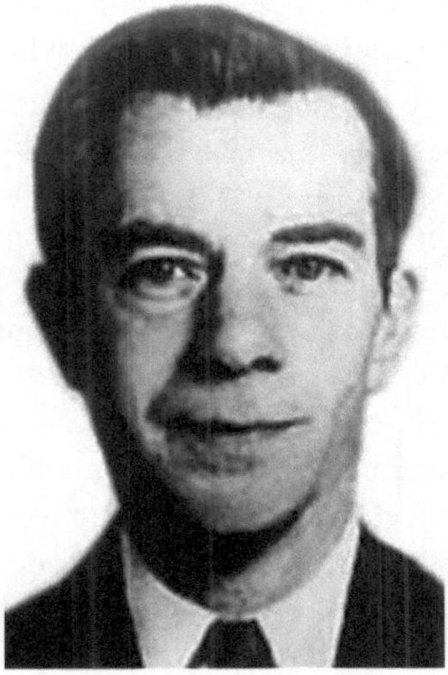

FIGURE 4.6 Willie Sutton

In 1952, Sutton was arrested for the last time. As prolific as he was as a bank robber, he was arguably even better at escaping. He managed to sneak out of some of the most heavily guarded prisons on four separate occasions. *Source:* Public domain.

often show why the explanandum (the thing we want to explain) *had* to happen somehow. In helping a man produce a child, a fertility doctor's discovery that the patient is unable to produce any semen explains his difficulties. It shows that, given his physiology, it would have been impossible for him to conceive a child with his partner without assistance. His infertility is not by chance, so to speak; rather, it is necessary given his physiology. Most contemporary philosophers are leery of metaphysical concepts such as necessity. What Hempel's model gives us is a way to understand why the explanandum *had* to occur without introducing any suspected metaphysical concepts. Instead, the explanandum was necessary because of logic. It was no surprise that the patient could not produce a child; he could not produce any semen. Hempel ingeniously replaces a vague concept of nomological necessity with a clear and precise concept of logical necessity.

In contrast to mind-independent theories of explanation, some philosophers argue that explanation is an essentially epistemic concept. To explain something is to render it comprehensible, demystified, or consistent with other accepted beliefs of the inquirer. Indeed, the etymology of the verb "to explain" can be traced back to its early meaning: to flatten or un-wrinkle something. To explain something thus has its roots in the act of making something plain to the inquirer. The exact perplexity that prompted a request of an explanation can clearly change from inquirer to inquirer. The classic story of Willie Sutton—the notorious bank robber of 40 years—being interviewed by reporter Mitch Ohnstad illustrates the relativity of explanation. Legend has it that Ohnstad asked Sutton upon his eventual arrest why he robbed banks: "Because that's where the money is," Sutton replied.

For Ohnstad, his interest was why Sutton *robbed* banks rather than not robbing at all; while Sutton took it as a question of why he robbed *banks* as opposed to some other targets.[8] The question "Why did Sutton rob banks?" can demand different explanations depending on exactly what perplexes the inquirer. Unlike mind-independent theories, an epistemic theory of explanation must make references to the inquirer's epistemic state.

These two theories of explanations represent two completely different approaches to understanding explanation, and the difference can have profound effects on how we do science. Recall the close connection between a hypothesis' explanatory power and its truth (that is, IBE). If the adequacy of an explanation is mind-independent, then whether a hypothesis explains the evidence would also be mind-independent. If one believes that citing the cause of the explanandum suffices for explaining it, then the connection between explanatory power and truth may be based on the objectivity of the causal story. A mind-independent theory of explanation provides a plausible justification for connecting truth and explanatory power. On the other hand, if explanations are epistemic, the connection between the two is much harder to establish. Suppose one believes that A explains B only if A scratches whatever epistemic itch that led the inquirer to ask, "Why B?" Finding epistemic solace need not have any connection with finding truths. We can believe in all sorts of hypotheses that remove the initial perplexity, and none of them has to be even approximately true. Indeed, drinking a bottle of wine often removes many perplexities we have about the world. The dichotomy between mind-independent and epistemic theories of explanation echoes the ambiguity in the goals of medicine: are we trying to find truths or are we trying to make our lives better? If medicine focuses only on improving our lives, whether the explanations are true is far less important. We infer a hypothesis because it best explains the observation; that is, the hypothesis best soothes our epistemic worries. Medicine tells (important) stories and we might even insist that these stories are "true"; nevertheless, the worth of the stories is ultimately grounded in their abilities to make us feel better both physically and epistemically.

4.5 A Case Against Mind-Independent Theories of Explanation

The most basic problem with all mind-independent theories of explanation is that they allow for the possibility that an explanation is adequate even if it fails to address the epistemic or psychological reason for the demand of the explanation in the first place. For mind-independent theorists, if the explanans stand in the proper relationship to the explanandum, we have an explanation. The inquirer can remain just as dumbfounded as before. This seems to be deeply counterintuitive.

Suppose we are at a public health roundtable and we are discussing why teenagers in a particular community have a higher rate of pregnancy. The answer "Because more of them are having unprotected sex" is "correct" in a sense. It is indeed true that the cause of pregnancy is generally unprotected sex. We might even be able to construct a Hempelian explanation to show why the rate of pregnancy in this community must be higher given certain biological laws of reproduction and facts about teenagers in the community. But these answers completely miss the point. What perplexes us is not that we are ignorant of how babies are made. We want to know why, given the context (e.g., there is competent sex education, free distribution of condoms, etc.), we still see an elevated rate of pregnancy.

The culprit, it seems, is that mind-independent theories of explanations are insensitive to the epistemic needs and contexts of the explanation. When we look for an explanation, we must know what it is about the observation that perplexes us. Bluntly citing a cause or folding the observation into a logical argument won't necessarily do the trick. We want to know why something happens, relative to what we already believe and know. This means that a proper theory of explanation must contain some epistemic facts about the inquirer.

A classic objection to Hempel's model can help illustrate the point. Known as the "flagpole objection," the example shows that plenty of arguments can easily satisfy his requirements of an adequate explanation and yet fail to explain. According to Hempel, we have an adequate explanation if we can logically deduce the explanandum from the explanans which contains at least one law of nature. Suppose I want to know why the shadow cast by a particular flag is X-feet long. A Hempelian explanation might look like this:

(1) The flagpole is Y-feet long.
(2) The angle of the sun is θ.
(3) According to the laws of trigonometry, if the length opposite of a triangle is Y and the angle of the hypotenuse is θ, then the length of the triangle is X. Therefore, the shadow is X-feet long.

So far, so good. But, of course, we can also derive the height of the flagpole using the length of the shadow and the angle of the sun. More ridiculous yet, we can derive the angle of the sun with the height of the flagpole and the length of the shadow. If it were this easy to explain the relative location of the sun in our sky, researching celestial mechanics would not take one beyond one's backyard with a flagpole!

A similar problem plagues causal theories of explanation. Having unprotected sex causes pregnancy but it doesn't explain why a specific community has a high teenage pregnancy rate. Being born is the leading cause of death, as philosophers joke, but it hardly explains why a perfectly healthy 25-year-old man dies suddenly. In order to identify the proper explanatory cause, we need to know what it was

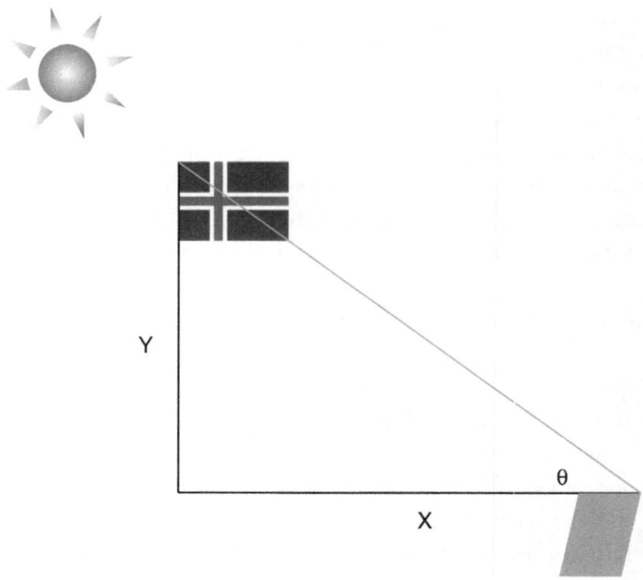

FIGURE 4.7 An Icelandic Flag Casting a Shadow

about observation that gave rise to the need for an explanation in the first place. And this must include the epistemic state of the inquirer.

Causal theorists are often aware of the contextual-relativity of citing *the* salient cause for an event. Perhaps we can import the same kind of flexibility into a causal account of explanation. The problem with this approach is that we would need to have a way to distinguish explanatory causes from non-explanatory ones. Among a plethora of causes, some of them are explanatory, and some not, for a given "why" question. How are we to tell them apart? Which one is the right one? A threat of circularity looms: we don't want to define a cause as explanatory just in case it explains. This would amount to the trivial definition that cause A explains effect B if and only if cause A explains effect B.

As an aside, medicine often implicitly assumes that citing a cause suffices for an explanation. To explain why a patient's cognitive functions are compromised, a clinician might point to his untreated syphilis as the cause of his general paresis. Hopefully, our brief discussion of causal theories of explanation should lead to a more cautious approach in declaring *the* cause of someone's health condition. Relative to certain interests, the cause of a patient's paresis might not be untreated syphilis per se, but rather his lack of access to adequate healthcare or failure to seek care. Talking about *the* cause would improperly privilege one set of epistemic concerns over all others. These kinds of blinders impose clinicians' values on their patients in a manner akin to past medical paternalism.

4.6 Epistemic Theories of Explanation

An epistemic theory of explanation pivots away from mind-independent analysis of explanations; instead, it takes the epistemic work that an explanation accomplishes as its defining quality. Most broadly, an adequate explanation is one that satisfies the epistemic needs of the inquirer which prompted the request for an explanation in the first place. In general, we ask for explanations because what we observe does not square with what we already believe. If we can make explicit what constitutes a proper resolution of the epistemic dissonance or disconnect, then we have an adequate epistemic theory of explanation.

Consider a fairly mundane medical puzzle. A patient presents symptoms of fatigue, depressive moods, changes in weight, and so on. Her previous physician had diagnosed hypothyroidism and recommended that she takes synthetic thyroid hormone. But in a follow-up visit, blood tests show that her thyroid level is in the normal range, and she is still exhibiting many of the symptoms of hypothyroidism. You suspect that she might be suffering from an unrelated mood disorder as well, and that could explain why her thyroid treatment has not significantly affected her depressive mood. The question "Why is the treatment for her hypothyroidism not improving her moods?" arises from a dissonance between your belief that a hypothyroid patient's moods should improve shortly after treatment begins and the observation that it has not. Abandoning the belief that the patient's hypothyroidism is the sole cause of her depressive mood resolves your dissonance. Of course, further treatment and observation will be needed to confirm that one is on the right diagnostic track. The point of this example is that in explaining an observation, we must first figure out what epistemic "woes" prompted the need for an explanation in the first place. Context sensitivity of this sort goes a long way to capture the explanatory relativity that we saw earlier. From finding the salient explanatory cause to subsuming an explanandum under the proper law, understanding the epistemic context of an explanation is indispensable in finding the right answer to a "why" question.

There are many ways an observation can fail to connect to our set of beliefs (or doxastic set, to borrow a philosophical term). It can be that an observation is "dangling." We simply don't know how we can connect what we see with what we already believe. Consider Alexander Fleming's observation that, upon returning from a two-week vacation, among his dirty petri dishes was one with samples of *Staphylococcus*. The mold that had grown in that dish formed a clear *Staphylococcus*-free ring. Fleming suspected that the mold contained a bacteria-killing substance, and we were well on our way to the discovery of penicillin. Fleming's observation did not explicitly conflict with what he believed; it dangled disconnected from everything else he believed. Identifying the anti-bacteria property of the mold provided an explanation for the observation and connected it to his doxastic set.

Alternatively, an observation might explicitly conflict with what the observer already believes. Whenever a promising therapeutic recommendation fails to improve a patient's condition, the care-provider is left wondering why. Given what she believes are true of her patient and of the therapeutic benefits of a treatment, the outcome is surprising. An explanation shows her how the conflict can be resolved. Perhaps a more careful look at her laboratory results shows that they were misread and that the diagnosis is likely incorrect. A proper explanation restores the coherence of her doxastic set and alleviates the dissonance that perplexed her in the first place.

There are a number of ways that an explanation can provide epistemic solace. Fitting an observation that had no apparent cause into one's broader causal picture of the world might be enough for an explanation. In this sense, citing the cause of an explanandum might be the right response to certain "why" questions. However, it is obvious that our explanatory perplexities are diverse, and citing a cause is not the only way we can explain. When Lois Lane wonders why Superman and Clark Kent have never been in the same room at the same time, explaining to her that they are one and the same person answers her question. An identification of two seemingly distinct things does not require that we cite any cause, but it can still be perfectly explanatory in some contexts.[9]

Epistemic theories of explanation can even offer some insights into our reaction to the flagpole objection. Van Fraassen (1980) tells a fictional scenario in which the height of a tower can be explained by the length of the shadow it casts. A chevalier fell madly in love with one of his maids. In a fit of jealousy, he murdered her. He built a tower of a certain height to ensure that it will always cast a shadow during sunset on the spot where he first fell in love with her. With enough contextual information, we can craft a scenario in which the perplexity can be removed by seemingly unusual explanations. While a mind-independent theory of explanation would have a tough time accommodating these unusual scenarios, an epistemic theory has little problem explaining them.

4.7 A Case Against Epistemic Theories of Explanation

Epistemic theories of explanation attempt to define explanatory adequacy on the basis of an explanation's ability to achieve certain epistemic gain. The main problem with all epistemic theories of explanation is that their proponents must be more precise about the concept of epistemic gain. Is it merely a matter of restoring logical consistency between the observation and our doxastic sets (likely too weak)? Moreover, we want to ensure that we distinguish epistemic gains that are explanatory from those that are not, and we need to do so in a non-question-begging manner. I might be puzzled by how the intricate human eye could have evolved gradually according to traditional Darwinian evolution. If an epistemic theory of explanation defines explanatory success in terms of the removal of the puzzlement, then what distinguishes a detailed evolutionary explanation from other non-explanatory means like a frontal lobotomy? Here, epistemic theories of explanation face a difficulty that is not unlike the one causal theories of explanation confront: how to specify the criteria for an adequate explanation without assuming a concept of explanation?

In addition, an epistemic theory of explanation might be too metaphysically weak, especially for those who rely on inference to the best explanation. An explanation is adequate, according to epistemic theories of explanation, if and only if the explanation achieves the proper epistemic ends. What is the relationship between achieving these ends and, say, truth? Why do we believe that the removal of perplexity means that the explanation is likely true? This is particularly problematic when we consider that our background beliefs can be radically false. We can live happily (with minimal epistemic dissonance) within a consistent set of false beliefs. An epistemic theory of explanation seems to undercut the connection between a hypothesis' explanatory power and its plausibility, and this raises serious questions about our reliance on IBE.[10]

Finally, if the aim of an explanation is to provide us with some epistemic solace, how do we make sense of our belief that explanations grant understanding (that goes beyond knowledge)? Epistemic theories of explanation seem to reduce the role of explanation to making us feel epistemically better. It is, at worst, the telling of comforting stories. Why should we care about epistemic solace from the point of view of science as a pursuit of discovering the nature of the universe? It feels good to have an explanation, but why is it the role of science to tell us stories that make us feel good? For those who question whether science can be done without the search for explanations, a quick reminder of Feynman's assessment that no one understands the whys of quantum mechanics might suffice. If science-without-explanation is good enough for physics, why is it not good enough for medicine? Fruitful and progressive scientific disciplines can exist while participants largely ignore the question of *why* things happen the way that they do.

We started this chapter by identifying many of the valuable things that we believe explanations can deliver. From learning about the nature of unobservable things to inferring the existence of laws of nature, from introducing theoretical entities that help guide direction of our research to providing narratives that relieve epistemic dissonances, the search for explanations is ubiquitous. Nonetheless, if we can conduct science and satisfy all our practical and even epistemic needs, freed from the constraints of explanations, should we still look for them? Does it matter why the patient suffers from a condition if at the end of the day we have the tools to make her feel better? In some respects, the questions here remind us of the great debate between Skinnerian behaviorists and their Freudian counterparts. If we can successfully treat and prevent the symptoms of diseases, does it really matter if we cannot identify the underlying causes? If we can eliminate all the symptomatic discomforts and mortal threats of, say, cancer, have we in fact found the cure for cancer? The question of whether explanations should play a role in medicine is thus twofold. Can we make research progress, diagnose, and treat adequately if we do not know the explanations of ailments and disabilities? And, if we can, why should medicine worry about explanations?

Notes

1 In physics, the search for explanations has largely been given a secondary importance. Take the problem of partial reflection. As one shines a beam of light at a plate of glass, a percentage of the light reflects from the surface. When the glass has an almost zero thickness, 0% reflects back. As the glass' thickness increases, the percentage of reflection increases. One would expect the reflection rate to increase proportionally, but experiments show that when the thickness hits a certain critical point, the rate of reflection decreases! Plotting out the reflection rates against the thickness of glass, we get not a straight proportional line but a sine wave. No one knows why this happens and, more importantly, the search for an explanation is less important for scientists than just figuring out the methods for calculating the behaviors of light in different mediums. As the great Richard Feynman warns his audience of their impending inability to understand his lectures on quantum electrodynamics, "The next reason that you might think you do not understand what I am telling you is, while I am describing to you *how* Nature works, you won't understand *why* Nature works that way. But you see, nobody understands that. I can't explain why Nature behaves in this peculiar way" (Feynman, 2014, p. 10).

2 In Molière's parody *The Imaginary Invalid*, a group of learned scholars asked a gifted student why opium induces sleep. The student replies that opium has a dormitive quality which explains why it induces sleep. Even with a fancy Latin name, the introduction of the hidden power "virtus dormitive" provides no real explanation for opium's ability to induce sleep. Another wonderful story illustrates the inadequacy of some explanations. A farmer listening to the radio in his home for the first time is amazed by how the performance of the Moscow Philharmonic can come into his home via the radio. He asks a scientist friend to explain it. "Imagine a very large dog with its tail in Moscow and its head in your home here in the country," the scientist says. "Now imagine that whenever someone pulls the tail in Moscow, the dog barks," he continues, "A radio works just like that except there is no dog."

3 In terms of research ethics, notice how far we have come. Semmelweis performed all these controlled experiments without the consent form or even awareness of his patients.

4 Semmelweis' hypothesis could not explain why we would find women contract childbed fever birthing at home, or an outbreak in his clinic *after* the handwashing regiment was adopted. Indeed, the puzzle led him to modify his theory at least twice more. He eventually settled on the hypothesis that morbid poison came not just from autopsies but from all decomposing animals.

5 For a fascinating look into the life of Semmelweis, see Nuland (2003). Although the lore of Semmelweis is well-known among medical professionals, historians of science, and philosophers of science, the orthodox story is likely too simplistic. For a more in-depth look at how Semmelweis theorized and the reasons why his professional community at large rejected his view, see the detailed research done by Tulodziecki (2013).

6 Like Semmelweis' experiments, Goldberger's trials contained gross ethical violations. The question of whether we should cite his work raises some serious ethical issues. The experiments performed by Nazi doctors in concentration camps, for instance, might provide invaluable data. But, citing these studies without qualms strikes me as morally questionable. Given how much of past medical research contains studies done unethically, a wholesale exorcizing of these trials would significantly impact the foundation of current research.

7 For a fantastic account of Goldberger's work on pellagra, see Alan Kraut's brilliant book *Goldberger's War: The Life and Work of a Public Health Crusader* (2004).

8 In his autobiography *Where the Money Was*, Sutton denies that he uttered his famous line; instead, he attributes it to the work of an enterprising and creative reporter. Sutton's example is doubly appropriate for our discussion of explanation. In medical school, students are often taught Sutton's Law, which tells clinicians to test for the most likely diagnosis first. Just as targeting banks makes for an efficient strategy for robberies, testing for the most likely pathology can save one's time and resources in diagnostics. Sutton's Law is simply a variation of inference to the best explanation.

9 Peter Lipton has written extensively on the epistemic work that explanations can do. (See Lipton, 2001, for example.)

10 One possible way to connect epistemic solace to truth is to adopt a coherence theory of truth that is favored by the American Pragmatists. If truth just means coherent beliefs, then an explanation's ability to generate coherence among our beliefs can thus lead us to truth. As with any coherence theory of truth, one worry is that truth becomes a relativistic notion. Because there are multiple ways to maintain consistency, what is true differs from one set of coherence beliefs to another. Giving up the objectivity of truth, for some philosophers, is a price too high to pay.

References

Clay, K., Schmick, E., Troesken, W., & National Bureau of Economic Research. (2017). The rise and fall of pellagra in the American South. *The Journal of Economic History, 79*(1), 32–62.

Feynman, R. P. (2014). *QED: The strange theory of light and matter.* Princeton, NJ: Princeton University Press.

Hampl, J. S., & Hampl, W. S. (1997). Pellagra and the origin of a myth: Evidence from European literature and folklore. *Journal of the Royal Society of Medicine, 90*(11), 636–639.

Kraut, A. M. (2004). *Goldberger's war: The life and work of a public health crusader.* New York, NY: Farrar, Straus and Giroux.

Lipton, P. (2001). What good is an explanation? In G. Hon & S. Rakover (Eds.), *Explanation* (pp. 43–59). The Netherlands: Springer Science+Business Media.

Mao, X. Q., Jia, X. F., Zhou, G., Li, L., Niu, H., Li, F. L., . . . Xu, N. (2011). Green tea drinking habits and gastric cancer in southwest China. *Asian Pacific Journal of Cancer Prevention, 12*(9), 2179–2182.

Nuland, S. (2003). *The doctors' plague: Germs, childhood fever, and strange story of Ignaz Semmelweis.* New York, NY: W. W. Norton.

Putnam, H. (1975). What is mathematical truth? *Mathematics, matter and method* (Vol. 1, pp. 60–78). Cambridge, UK: Cambridge University Press.

The UK ECT Review Group. (2003). Efficacy and safety of electroconvulsive therapy in depressive disorders: A systematic review and meta-analysis. *The Lancet, 361*(9360), 799–808. doi:https://doi.org/10.1016/S0140-6736(03)12705-5

Tulodziecki, D. (2013). Shattering the myth of Semmelweis. *Philosophy of Science, 80*(5), 1065–1075.

van Fraassen, B. (1980). *The scientific image* (1st ed.). New York, NY: Clarendon Press.

5

PROBABILITIES IN MEDICINE

5.1 Varieties of Chances

In the last two chapters, we looked at the nature of evidence and explanation. Both are intimately connected to the concept of probabilities. An observation is a piece of positive evidence if it raises the probability of certain hypotheses, for instance. For inference to the best explanation, a hypothesis' ability to explain a set of observations makes the hypothesis more likely to be true. Probability and its cousins, likelihood and confidence, are so fundamental to scientific reasoning that it is fitting to end our trio of conceptual discussions with a close examination of how we should understand probabilistic claims.

Like many empirical sciences, medicine converses in the language of probability. The lifetime probability of developing lung cancer for a male Canadian smoker is 172/1,000. The 10-year survival rate of a 64-year-old who suffered from heart failure is 26.7%. Parents who are both carriers of the Tay-Sachs genes have a 25% chance of conceiving a child with the disease. Probabilistic claims are indispensable in helping a patient make the appropriate therapeutic choice, in shaping public health policies to mitigate health risks, in continuation of clinical trials, and countless other examples. At the same time, our understanding of probability is hardly crystal clear. Suppose we learn that 15 out of 100 subjects in a study developed certain undesirable side-effects from a specific treatment. How should an individual who is considering the same treatment interpret this information? This question goes deeper than a question of how we translate clinical data to bedside applications. It touches on fundamental questions of what probabilistic claims actually mean. In this example, does the 15/100, or 15%, reflect the person's objective chance of developing these side-effects? What does objective chance mean? Does it mean if there are 100 similar individuals, 15 of them *will* experience the side-effects? Or, does it mean we should *expect* 15 of them will experience the side-effects, but that there is no guarantee that 15 will? How confident should I be about this prediction?

Alternatively, does 15% tell me how I should set my subjective confidence level (credence or degree of belief)? Credence often serves as guide to rational decision-making. It would be irrational, for instance, for me to act as if the chance of the side-effects is zero. Likewise, it would be irrational for me to overweigh the risk and treat it as a virtual guarantee. All calculations of expected utility (some believe to be the basis of rational decision-making) take into consideration the likelihood of outcomes. We need to understand what likelihood means if we are to justify our reliance on expected utility calculation in, say, determining public health policies.

It is important to note that our discussion here is less about the statistical competence of healthcare providers and patients in general. Their inadequacies are well reported and studied. In an eye-opening piece, Casscells, Schoenberger, and Graboys (1978) attempted to evaluate healthcare providers' competency in understanding laboratory test results. They posed the following question to 60 people, made up of physicians, medical students, and house officers (residents), from four Harvard Medical School teaching hospitals:

> If a test to detect a disease whose prevalence is 1/1000 has a false positive rate of 5%, what is the chance that a person found to have a positive result actually has the disease, assuming you know nothing about the person's symptoms or signs?

If the test is perfectly sensitive, the correct answer should be 1.96%.[1] The good news is that if you got it wrong, you are in very good company. The vast majority of respondents gave an incorrect answer, with almost half answering "95%"—astonishingly, a full 48X overestimation.

Some critics of the study have suggested that the Casscells et al. results stemmed from poor biostatistics training in past medical education. But Manrai, Bhatia, Strymish, Kohane, and Jain (2014) repeated the study recently and selected subjects with similar backgrounds as in the first study. Depressingly, their findings differ little from those of Casscells et al. (with 44% answering "95%"). Apparently the "improvements" in biostatics education in the past 40 years have done little to better equip healthcare providers in understanding statistical information.

The failure to understand health statics among laypersons, journalists, and policy-makers can be equally if not more distressing. In 1995, the U.K.'s Committee on Safety of Medicines warned that the use of third-generation birth-control pills that contain gestodene or desogestrel have a risk for venous thromboembolism that is twice as high as that of earlier generations. Thousands of women stopped taking oral contraceptives leading to a significant increase of abortions and unplanned births. However, if one digs deeper into the statistics, the risk of a woman developing venous thromboembolism without being on birth-control pills is 1 in 7,000, while for women on the birth-control pills, the risk is 2 in 7,000. Although the relative risk was in fact twice as high, the absolute risk of developing venous thromboembolism was still remarkably small. Given the harm caused by the abrupt cessation of oral birth-control, a mis-comprehension of the statistics (and the warning issued) led to poor public health and clinical decisions.

To be sure, one of the reasons why needless screenings and tests are carried out stems from the culture of defensive medicine. Care-providers worry that if do not order tests and their patients develop a condition later, they could become legally liable. This "more-is-better" approach not only drives up medical expenses, it also creates fertile ground for useless interventions, harmful biopsies, and needless psychological strain. Without placing a statistical result in the proper context, one can be left with a wildly inaccurate understanding of one's health, the harm and benefit of a treatment, and the wisdom of life-choices.[2]

Perhaps, with better education in biostatistics, patients and healthcare providers can more properly interpret statistical claims. Nevertheless, even with perfect knowledge of the mathematics of statistics, there are some fundamental challenges regarding how we ought to understand statistical claims. These problems are philosophical in nature, and no amount of mathematical training can solve them. In this chapter, we will explore three of the most common ways philosophers have attempted to understand probabilistic claims. We will discuss their philosophical foundations and the problems that confront them, especially in relation to how they should inform our decision-making.

5.2 Frequency Distribution: The Report of Brute Facts

Perhaps the most obvious interpretation of probability claims is that they report frequency or distribution of a sample. In Manrai et al.'s example earlier, we notice that 27 out of 61 subjects surveyed came up with the incorrect answer of "95%." Simple division then tells us that the percentage of healthcare providers who offered that answer is 44%. This number, per se, reports the portion of individuals answering "95%" over the total number of subjects. Similarly, we might hear that the infant mortality rate (death within the first year) in the United States is 5.8 per 1,000 live births (ranked 33 out of 44 countries among the Organization for Economic Co-operation and Development). To derive this number, epidemiologists collect data from across the U.S., identify the number of deaths within the first year of birth, and divide the number over the total number of life-births over the same period. Reducing the denominator to a net 1,000 number gives us a rough idea of the percentage of infants' deaths. It is akin to looking into a box of Legos blocks, and concluding that 26% of them are green by dividing the total of green blocks over the total number of blocks. Most medical research follows this methodology when deriving a probabilistic conclusion: it reports the general distribution of a sample observed.

Given the fact that frequency distribution merely states the brute numbers and fractions of what we have observed, they cannot account for all types of probabilistic claims. For instance, if I claim that the probability that there are extraterrestrial lifeforms somewhere in the universe is virtually 100%, I am certainly not making a numeric report of observation of how many universes I have observed and what fraction of them have extraterrestrial lifeforms. For one thing, I have not actually seen an extraterrestrial lifeform. Moreover, I am also not claiming that I have managed to travel across parallel universes (alas) and looked for extraterrestrial lifeforms in each of them. Single-case examples of this sort present problems for a straightforward interpretation of probability claims as frequency distributions alone. As such, frequency distribution represents just one way to interpret them.

As plain reports of observations, frequency distributions can be of great use. If I plan to lobby the U.S. Senate, knowing that 51% of senators are Republicans is helpful. Similarly, learning that the atmosphere of Mars contains only 0.14% oxygen certainly affects my plans to travel there. Unlike the Senate example, however, our Mars example does not involve the sampling of *all* of Mars' atmosphere. We had to extrapolate the overall composition from the limited observations we have made. When we learn that about 75% of Harvard-affiliated healthcare providers sampled failed the probability quiz, we generalize that information and conclude that 75% of *all* clinicians cannot do basic statistical analyses. The real power of frequency distribution lies in its ability to extrapolate a broader conclusion from the limited observation. These probabilistic reports tell us not just what we have observed, but they also aim to let us make broader generalizations about things that we have not.

Going from a limited sample to a general claim is, of course, the very nature of inductive reasoning. The Scottish philosopher David Hume famously raised a fundamental problem with justifying our reliance on induction.[3] According to Hume, to demonstrate that induction is justified, we need to show that induction, as a method of reasoning, is reliable; that is, induction produces largely true beliefs. There are two possible ways we can do this. We can either show that "Induction is reliable" is a conceptual truth on a par with "Triangles have three sides." Or, we can show that it is an empirical truth like "Wombats are mammals." Obviously, "Induction is reliable" is not a conceptual truth because it is possible that induction is *not* reliable. There is no inherent reliability in the *concept* of induction. Perhaps we can show that induction is reliable because of its stellar past performance. Whenever we look to see if induction delivers true beliefs, we note that it has largely done so. Induction has a great track record, so to speak. The problem with using the past reliability of induction to justify its overall reliability is that the justification is itself an inductive argument. In other words, we are using induction to justify induction! It is like asking your shifty friend if he is lying to you. His declaration "Of course not!" would bring little confidence

Using frequency distribution of past observations to project claims about what we have not observed runs immediately into Hume's problem of induction. Yet,

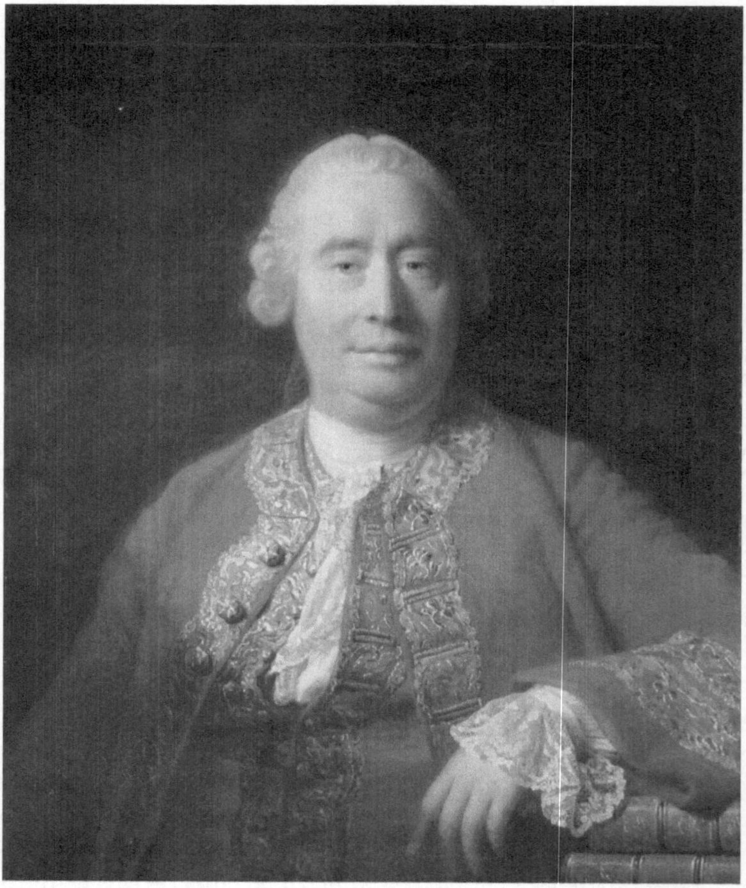

FIGURE 5.1 A 1766 Portrait of David Hume by Allan Ramsay

In 1999, *Sunday Times* surveyed academics and opinion formers to select the Scot of the Millennium. Hume not only beat out his close friend Adam Smith, he also topped Robert Burns, and Alexander Fleming. During his lifetime, however, Hume was unlucky in life as he was in love. Due to his reputation of being an atheist, Hume was twice denied an academic post at University of Edinburgh. His publications made little splash and he called their receptions "deadborn from the press." Meanwhile, he was madly infatuated with Hippolyte de Saujon, the wife of the Comte de Boufflers and mistress of the Prince de Conti. When the Comte de Boufflers finally died, Hippolyte de Saujon singularly focused her attention on marrying the prince, leaving Hume in the role of a platonic advisor. Never married and professionally marginalized, Hume died with no inkling that his ideas would help shape the trajectory of Western thoughts for centuries. Indeed, his final work, *Dialogues Concerning Natural Religion*, published after his death, is considered by many as an intellectual predecessor to Charles Darwin's theory of natural selection. Hume serves as great inspiration during our more disillusioned moments. *Source:* Public domain.

without the ability to project, frequency distribution is, at most, interesting as reported observations only. Indeed, if we restrict probabilistic claims to nothing but reports of past observations, clinical research would have no way of using the information to guide future clinical and research practices. The entire domain of medical sciences arguably rests on being able to justify induction. Philosophy has yet to find a satisfactory response to Hume's problem. The gravity of his challenge to the rationality of induction has led many philosophers to conclude that the Humean dilemma is the human dilemma.

Another basic problem with the frequency interpretation of probability is the fact that there are multiple ways we can categorize our samples. Depending on which description we choose, we can get radically different probabilities. Known as the "reference class problem," this challenge is taken by most philosophers as fatal to the entire frequency approach.[4] Consider a straightforward clinical question: what is the probability that Brad will live until he is 80? Suppose as a 50-year-old American male, he has a 57% chance. However, if we categorize him as a two-pack-a-day white male smoker, his chances are now at 34%. Imagine that we gather mortality data of people who have lived in Cincinnati for more than five years, have visited Hawaii at least twice, and have had ferrets as pets. It turns out that 82% of this unique cohort, which Brad is a member of, live to 80. Which probability is right? To answer that question, we have to identify the "correct" way to describe Brad. We know what his probability is if we describe him as Brad-the-smoker or Brad-the-former-Cincinnati-resident-who-went-to-Hawaii-twice-and-has-a-pet-ferret. But the initial question asks, "What is the probability that *Brad* lives to 80?" It doesn't ask for the conditional probability of Brad-as-X or Brad, given X. If we think there is an answer to the unconditional probability question, then these conditionalized probabilities are of no use. Frequency interpretation of probabilities that require us to put our samples in certain categories (e.g., as smokers) would thus never be able to give us an answer to the unconditional probability question.

One might think that we can avoid the problem by categorizing Brad as narrowly as possible. He is a white American male who is 50. He smokes two packs a day, lived in Cincinnati for five years, has been to Hawaii twice, and owns a ferret. If we slice our collective samples to this narrower class, then we will have a more accurate description of Brad. The hope is that if we keep doing this, we can eventually get a probability answer for *the* Brad. The problem with this approach is that there are infinitely many ways we can narrow Brad. Brad also lives in a house built in the 1910s. He drives an imported car and likes to go rock-climbing. As we continue to narrow down the sample with more categories, our sample size decreases. Eventually, we arrive at the absurd conclusion that the correct description of Brad picks Brad out and no one else. A sample size of one is hardly the stuff of inductive confidence.

We might also be tempted to exclude certain categories as clinically irrelevant. The fact that Brad has 17 red t-shirts should have no bearing on his life-expectancy. Indeed, we might even dismiss any possible statistical correlations (if there are any) between the ownership of t-shirts and longevity, because the former simply has nothing to do with the latter. Here, we find ourselves in the unfortunate and familiar territory of determining just what makes a mere regularity a universal law. Our discussion of Goodman's New Problem of Induction in Chapter 3 should dispel any faint hope that we can straightforwardly justify this commonsensical response.

5.3 The Principle of Indifference, or How Gambling Gave Us Modern Statistics

Before we proceed to discuss the other interpretations of probability, there is a general problem with how we "slice" up probabilistic space in general. Consider someone who wants to know the odds of rolling a six on a typical six-sided die. He slices up the probability space in the following manner: one to five represents one outcome and six represents the other. Furthermore, he assigns two equal probabilities to each outcome; that is, 0.5 for one to five and 0.5 for six. This is obviously an incorrect assignment of probability. The outcome one to five is clearly far more likely than the outcome six. In fact, it is five times more likely. How are we to explain to him his incorrect initial partitioning of the probability space? The 18th century French mathematician Pierre-Simone Laplace outlines the Principle of Indifference that continues to serve as the basis of modern probability, and it shows us why the division of probability space in this example is incorrect. The Principle, as outline in his 1812 *A Philosophical Essay on Probabilities*, goes as follows:

> The theory of chance consists in reducing all the events of the same kind to a certain number of cases equally possible, that is to say, to such as we may be equally undecided about in regard to their existence, and in determining the number of cases favorable to the event whose probability is sought. The ratio of this number to that of all the cases possible is the measure of this probability, which is thus simply a fraction whose numerator is the number of favorable cases and whose denominator is the number of all the cases possible.
>
> *(Chapter II)*

When we first learn of probability as children, we were likely taught a variation of this principle. There are three doors, one of them has a goat behind it, what are the odds that if I randomly open a door, there would be a goat there? The answer 1/3 comes easily with an almost reflexive application of the Principle of Indifference. The mistake of slicing the probability space in the die example above is precisely that the one-to-five and six are not the same kind. As such, the Principle of Indifference tells us that we should not assign the same probability to them.

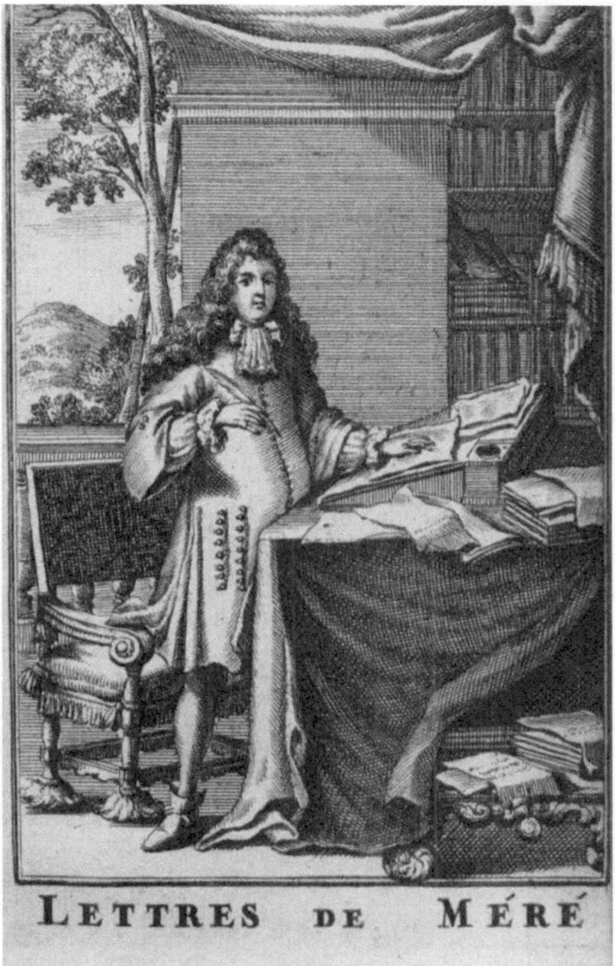

FIGURE 5.2 Antoine Gombaud

A frontispiece in volume two of a collection of speeches, *Les Oeuvres de Monsieur le Chevalier de Méré* (1692), by Antoine Gombaud (1607–1684). Although not of royal descent, the writer and professional gambler first used the title "Chevalier de Méré" for a sympathetic character in his writing. He later adopted the name in real life. The Chevalier calculated incorrectly the probability of rolling two sixes in a series of 24 rolls. The error proved costly and he solicited the help of Blaise Pascal and Pierre de Fermat to solve the problem. Their collaboration led to the development of formal probability theories that formed the foundation for Laplace's work.

On further and more careful reflection, the Principle appears to contain some basic problems. Laplace tells us that all events of the "same kind" should receive equal probability assignments. The six sides of a die, for instance, belong to the same kind and, therefore, they should each be assigned the same probability (with the sum adding up to 1). This diagnosis, however, faces a new problem; namely, how can we tell if two things belong to the same kind with respect to probability? After all, the six sides of a die are not identical. Indeed, if construed narrowly enough, no two objects are identical. We strongly believe that differences like microscopic scratches on a die surface do not preclude two die faces from belonging to the same type. But what about the different pips (dots on a die's face)? What if one of the faces were painted differently?

Suppose we roll a die a great number of times, perhaps 1,000. Should the outcome be equivalent to *the* probability of the die's behaviors when rolled? For instance, if one side comes up far more frequently than 1 in 6, should we conclude that there must be some physical differences between that side and the other sides such that they no longer belong to the same kind? If we follow this route, then the Principle of Indifference no longer serves any purpose. We do not antecedently slice up each of the probabilistic outcomes that belong to the same type and assign them the same probability. The case of assigning one-to-five and six equal probability would not be mistaken (at least not until we start rolling). As we have seen, identifying probability with frequency distribution raises a host of philosophical problems. It also leads to some fairly counterintuitive consequences and technical problems. For example, two people who roll the same die 1,000 times are very likely not going to get the same outcome. Do we want to say that there are *two* probabilities for the same die? One for you and one for me? How long are we supposed to roll before it becomes sufficient to establish the probability? If we suggest that we consider the outcomes "at the limit," how do we know what those are without already presupposing the Principle of Indifference?

The alternative is to specify exactly what makes two outcomes belong to the same kind. Obviously, some physical differences matter and some physical differences don't. Ideally, we want to have a definition that fills in the right side of this statement:

> A and B belong to *the same kind* if and only if their physical differences are. . . .

Since "belong to the same kind" just means having the same probability outcome, according to the Principle of Indifference, the task is really filling in the right side of the following:

> A and B have *the same probabilities* if and only if their physical differences are. . . .

What are we to put in place of the ellipses? The answer "A and B have the same probabilities if and only if their physical differences do not amount to a difference in probability" would obviously be circular and trivial. So, we want the right side to say something that does not include references to identical probabilities. In essence, we need to know what physical criterion has to be satisfied for two outcomes to be equally probable. And, we want to specify this in language without referencing probability. The hope of successfully completing this project seems dim. And, without that answer, it would be impossible for us to specify antecedently what constitutes the same class or, to be put it differently, whether two outcomes should in fact be assigned the same probability.

One might be tempted to rely on past knowledge to determine what physical characteristics affect probability outcomes. For instance, we believe that the color of a die face makes no difference (unless, one side is painted with particularly heavy paint). We believe this because, in the past, we have observed many instances where the color of the object did not affect its physical behaviors when tossed. This approach, however, merely pushes the problem back. How were we able to derive the past knowledge? If we appeal to past frequency distributions, then the Principle of Indifference is again useless and we are once again stuck with the problems that confront frequency distribution theory of probability. If we appeal to some knowledge that did not come from frequency distribution (e.g., some past applications of the Principle of Indifference), then we enter a regress. What is justifying our confidence that *those* outcomes are equally probable? In either case, there seems to be no easy way to save the Principle of Indifference.

Although this brief discussion might appear to be highly abstract and technical, its relevance to medical research is salient. Consider a study that groups together 200 subjects for a drug trial dividing them evenly between an active arm and a no-treatment control arm. Each subject is taken to have equal probability of responding to the drug (once we have controlled for all the "relevant" confounders). Suppose a large subgroup of subjects is particularly sensitive to the experimental drug; perhaps, the drug is twice as effective for them. When the trial ends, the researchers learn that 40 out of the 100 subjects in the active arm have improved significantly (compared to 20 from the control arm). If the researchers conclude that the drug is 20% more effective than no treatment, the conclusion would be incorrect, since there was a confounder among the subjects that the researchers missed. The sample was, in fact, biased. If, say, among the 40 subjects who responded positively, 35 of them turned out to be from the idiosyncratic subgroup, then the percentage of the general population (and tested subjects) who would benefit from the drug would be lower. The researchers had erroneously assumed that the subjects were all roughly equivalent; specifically, that they had the same chances of responding to the drug.

Perhaps by increasing our sample size and conducting more replication studies, we can rule out the presence of unknown confounders. The difficulty with this solution is that for any sample, we can *always* group together characteristics of a subgroup that are statistically correlated with certain experimental outcomes. The fact that all subjects with last names longer than seven letters happen to perform better strikes most of us as a fun coincidence and not evidence of a biased sample. This confidence, however, rests on our ability to distinguish accidental correlations from nomological regularities. As we saw earlier, there is no obvious way for us to do that. The application of the Principle of Indifference thus presupposes a solution to Goodman's New Problem of Induction. Any experimental setup that relies on this principle to assign initial probabilities would therefore be saddled with a heavy philosophical burden.

5.4 Subjective Probability: Do You Feel Lucky?

What makes the Principle of Indifference so attractive is that it promises a way to assign probabilities to different outcomes before we start any testing trials. In philosophy, we call it an *a priori* assignment of initial probabilities; that is, an assignment of initial probabilities without using any empirical evidence. As we conduct empirical trials, we might revise our initial assignments in light of new evidence. The Principle of Indifference thus gives us a starting point. The problems associated with it come from our need to have a way to justify our initial probability assignments. If we can abandon this commitment, however, we might rid ourselves of the philosophical difficulties with the Principle of Indifference.

I believe that $2+2=4$. I also believe that it is not going to rain tomorrow. Nevertheless, I am more confident that $2+2=4$ than that it is not going to rain tomorrow. I can represent my levels of confidence with numbers; e.g., I am 99% certain that $2+2=4$, and I am 72% certain that it will not rain tomorrow. Subjective theories of probability treat probability statements as reflections of individuals' confidence levels. When a clinician says that there is an 80% chance that her patient's conditions will improve, according to subjective theories, she is expressing her subjective confidence or, in philosophical jargon, her credence.

The more radical version takes the assignment of initial probability as not guided by any constraints short of some basic requirements. These requirements might include principles such as $P(A) + P(\sim A) = 1$, or the sum of the probability of A and the probability of not-A is equal to one. But, short of some basic requirements, one can assign whatever probability value to an event one sees fit.[5]

Unlike those relying on frequency distribution or the Principle of Indifference, there is no philosophical demand to justify one's assignments of initial probabilities (short of some notion of coherence). If I wanted to assign the odds of one coming up on a six-sided die as 1/3, it is entirely permissible according to the subjectivist theory of probability. The flexibility of subjective probability nicely captures how we ordinarily respond to new information. For instance, suppose I am a firm believer in the therapeutic benefits of a chemotherapy protocol; say I assign a 90% chance that a certain chemotherapy protocol would improve a patient's condition. If I read a study that shows the contrary outcome, depending on how rigorous I believe the study was conducted, I might lower my confidence level to perhaps 88%. It is still high and high enough for me to continue recommending it. On the other hand, for someone who starts out with a lower confidence level (e.g., 64%), a drop in 2% might lead him to change his mind about the therapeutic benefits of the protocol. Whether additional evidence "tips the scale" depends not only on where the tipping points are for each of us, but also on our initial probability. A firm theist might be troubled by an argument for atheism, but she might not be troubled enough to become an atheist. Subjective probability does a wonderful job of explaining why two clinicians can look at the same study and come to different but equally rational conclusions about the therapeutic benefits of a treatment. Probability, according to the subjectivists, is a measurement of confidence often relative to information we have. The connection between the two can best be illustrated with the classic Monty Hall Paradox.

The paradox is modeled on the game show *Let's Make a Deal* hosted by Monty Hall. A contestant is given a chance to choose one of three doors to open. Behind one of the doors is the grand prize. There is a lousy prize behind the other two doors; for example, a goat. After the contestant has chosen a door, Hall opens *one* of the remaining doors and shows that it contains a goat. The contestant is then given a chance to switch her initial choice with the remaining unopened door. Does it alter her chance of winning the grand prize if she switches? Mathematicians had thought that the contestant's decision to switch makes no difference to her chance of winning the prize. Indeed, when the paradox was published in Parade Magazine in 1990 in Marilyn vos Savant's column, she received thousands of letters from learned mathematicians criticizing her answer that the contestant's odds of winning would go up if she switches. The obvious intuition for not switching is this: when the contestant was presented with the three doors, her odds of winning the grand prize were one in three (assuming the Principle of Indifference!). When Hall shows her a goat behind one of the doors, her chance of winning couldn't possibly have changed. Nothing "physical" has been altered in the setup; the prize has not been moved. If her chance of winning was 1/3, it should remain 1/3.

The appeal of switching, however, is a bit harder to grasp. To understand it, we need to keep in mind that Hall did not open the empty door by chance. He *knew* that the door he was opening would reveal nothing. This additional piece of information tells the contestant something about the odds of her having picked the correct door. We can map out her choices this way (Figure 5.4):

Suppose the contestant picks door 1 (where the grand prize sits). Hall opens one of the remaining doors (say door 2) and the contestant switches her choice. Hall opens door 3 and she loses. Suppose the contestant picks door 2. Hall opens door 3. The remaining door is the grand prize; she switches and she wins. Finally, suppose the contestant picks door 3. Hall opens door 2. Switching to door 1 once again leads her to the grand prize. Therefore, adopting the switching strategy would increase her chance of winning the grand prize from 1/3 (the staying strategy) to 2/3. What is so remarkable about this example is that nothing physical has changed in terms of the prize and the door in front of it. If the probability of a prize behind a given door is based only on the physical properties of the door and the prize, then the probability that the prize is behind door that she has

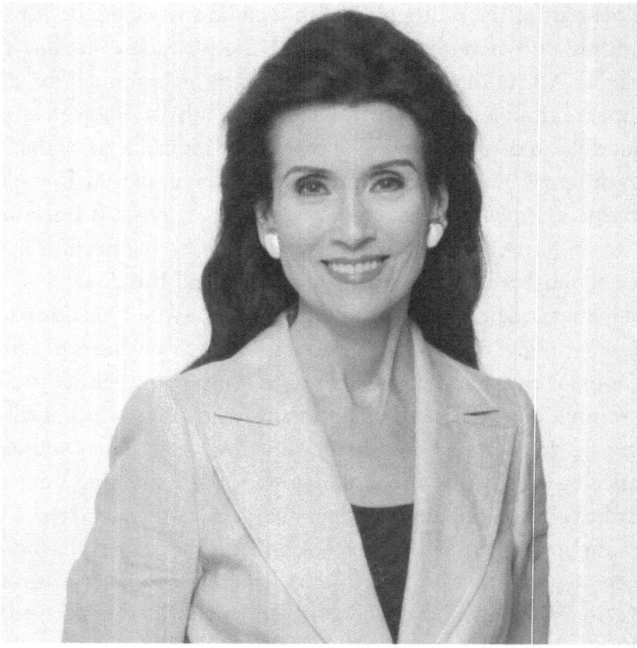

FIGURE 5.3 Marilyn vos Savant

Marilyn vos Savant is a national columnist, an author, and an executive at Jarvik Heart, Inc. (a maker of artificial hearts). She has also been recognized as having the highest IQ for both childhood and adult scores by the Guinness Book of World Records. *Source:* Image from www.flickr.com/photos/156235789@N02/41959101350 for Parade Magazine by Ethan Hill.

picked should remain the same. By opening a loser door, Monty Hall provides the contestant with more information. The improved probability of the switching strategy essentially means that the contestant has more evidence that the other door has the grand prize (as opposed to the door she initially chose). In this sense, probability seems to be a measurement not of some objective physical state of the world but of our subjective degree of confidence. Indeed, if Monty Hall opens both doors and reveals that they are both losers, it would be ridiculous to maintain that the contestant's chance of having chosen the correct door remains the same as before. Chance, it seems, is a matter of ignorance.

We can accentuate the importance knowledge plays in the Monty Hall Paradox by imagining a scenario in which Hall *doesn't know* which door has the grand prize and randomly opens a door which happens to be the goat prize. In this scenario, would it make sense for the contestant to switch? Consider her choices again (See Table 5.1).

Suppose she picks door 1 and Hall randomly opens a door 2. She switches and she loses. But since Hall's choice was random (he has no idea where the grand prize actually is), we need to consider the possibility that Hall opens door 3. Since door 2 also contains the goat prize, by switching, the contestant loses as well.

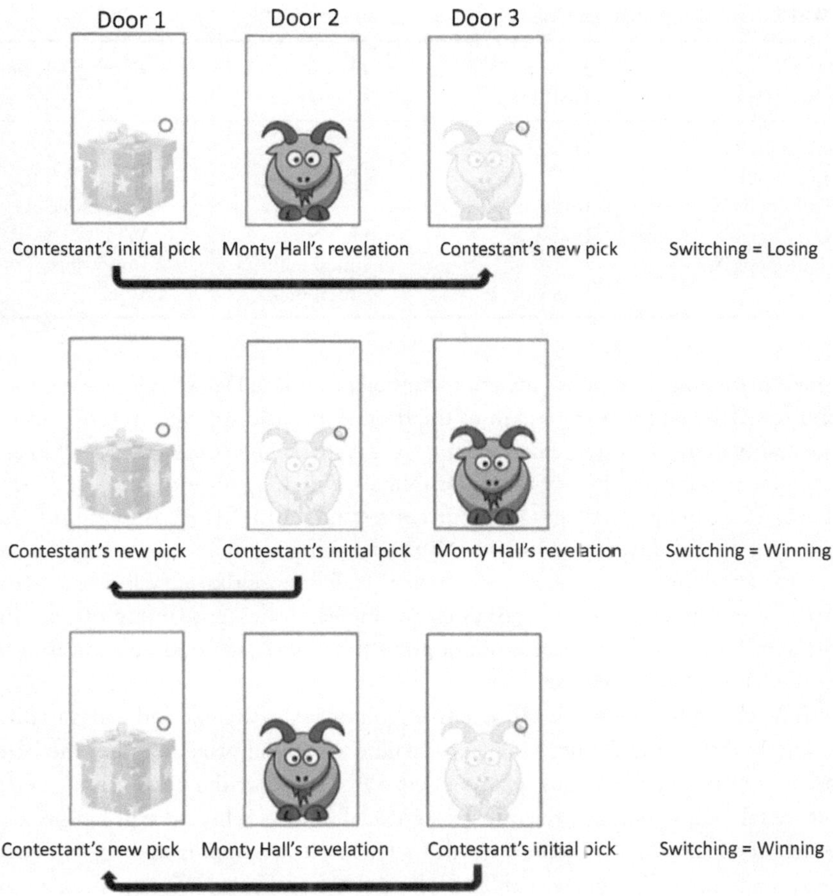

FIGURE 5.4 Monty Hall

If the contestant starts out with door 2, the outcome is a bit more complicated. Again, the question is whether the contestant's odds of winning would go up if she switches after Hall reveals a goat. In this variation, Hall does not know where the grand prize is; therefore, his opening of the goat door is due to sheer luck. Suppose Hall opens door 1 and inadvertently reveals the grand prize. Given that we want to know whether switching improves the odds *after* Hall has opened a goat door, Hall's opening door 1 and showing the grand prize would have precluded the setup. In other words, if Hall had opened door 1, we would not be in the scenario in which the contestant picks a door and Hall opens a goat door. Since we are interested in knowing the probability of switching if the latter scenario occurs, Hall's opening door 1 would have prevented the scenario from taking place. Thus, we can ignore that possibility as moot. On the other hand, suppose Hall opens door 3, the contestant's switching to door 1 will win her the

TABLE 5.1 Monty Hall paradox With Hall's ignorance

Door 1 *Grand Prize*	*Door 2* *Goat Prize*	*Door 3* *Goat Prize*	*Result of switching*
Initial pick	Hall opens		Lose
Initial pick		Hall opens	Lose
Hall opens **X**	Initial pick		Impossible
	Initial pick	Hall opens	Win
Hall opens **X**		Initial pick	Impossible
	Hall opens	Initial pick	Win

grand prize. Finally, suppose the contestant picks door 3. Hall cannot open door 1 and reveal a goat for reasons akin to the door 2 scenario. So we can rule out that possibility as moot as well. Hall opens door 2 instead. The contestant switches and wins the grand prize. In 2 of the 4 possibilities, switching leads to the grand prize. Thus, the switching strategy gives our contestant a 50% chance of winning. But, since the probability of winning for NOT switching is just 1−P(switching), it too is 50%. Therefore, switching for cases where Hall does not know where the grand prize is and merely guesses right does not increase one's probability of winning the grand prize. Switching does not improve the contestant's odds in this variation of the Monty Hall Paradox.

The difference between the original Monty Hall Paradox and our variation is simply that in the former Hall *knows* where the grand prize is and in the latter he does not. In order to answer the question of whether the contestant is better off switching, we actually need to know if Hall knows where the grand prize is. A Monty Hall who saunters onto the set completely unprepared for the day's show and happens to guess correctly where the grand prize is by opening a goat door provides no useful information for the contestant. As such, his opening the door does not change my probability of winning (if I switch). Probabilities, in this case, behave a great deal like measurements of confidence and information. The contestant's confidence in the location of the grand prize changes in light of new information (Hall's opening the door). And the evidence has to be epistemically special: Hall's opening a door is only useful if he *knew* where the goat was.

When there is no evidence guiding our confidence, subjectivism tells us that we can assign whatever probability that we would like. If we are particularly risk-averse, we might assign a high probability of an undesirable outcome. Alternatively, we might indulge in some wishful thinking and surmise that an outcome is highly probable. There is nothing that constrains our initial assignments of subjective probabilities.[6]

One might worry that a subjective interpretation is too permissive and offers little use in empirical application. It would surely be ridiculous for a patient to see two different doctors and receive two radically different but equally valid probabilistic answers to the question "What are my odds of surviving my ailment?" What good are probability claims if anyone can say any number and be as "correct" as another? The key to providing some objectivity to subjective probabilities rests on the notion of updating. Subjective probability theorists argue that there are rigorous algorithms that tell us how to revise our probability in light of new evidence. One of the most well-known and widely adopted algorithms is Bayes' Theorem. In fact, it is so entrenched that subjective probability theories are often called Bayesian Probability.

An 18th century English mathematician and minister, Thomas Bayes proposed a formula to calculate inferential logic. His eponymous theorem was published posthumously by his literary executor, the philosopher and mathematician Richard Price, in 1763. In its modern form, Bayes' Theorem says:

$$P(A/B) = P(A) \times P(B/A)/P(B)$$

To put it in plain English, the probability of event A given B is the probability of A multiplied by the probability of B given A divided by the probability of B. When Bayesians use the term "probability of A given B," they mean something like the probability of A in light of some other claim B. The probability that I roll six given I have already rolled an even number would be the probability of rolling a six, assuming I had already rolled an even number. The answer would thus be 1/3. In clinical medicine, the probability of a patient having lung cancer goes up if he is a regular smoker. This idea of probability of something given something else is often called "conditional probability." Although Bayes' Theorem appears technical and cryptic, its basic rationale is easy to grasp.

Let's return to the probability question posed by Manrai et al. that we introduced earlier. The specifics of the question are: disease D occurs in 1 in 1,000 individuals "in the wild," and a test that detects D is perfectly accurate (that is, if someone has D, the test would reveal it 100% of the time), but it has a false-positive rate of 5%. What is the probability that individual S has D if S is tested positive for D? For this question, A would be "S has D" and B would be "S is tested positive for D." We can now plug in the numbers using Bayes' Theorem and determine the probability that S has the disease given S has tested positive for the disease.

$$P(\text{S has D/S is tested positive for D}) = 0.001 \times 1 \,/\, \left[(0.001 \times 1) + (0.999 \times 0.05)\right]$$

The numerator of the equation is easy to understand. P(S has D) is just the probability that S has the disease in the wild and we were told that the probability is 1 in 1,000. P(S is tested positive for D/S has D) is the probability that a test would reveal the disease if S has the disease and we stipulate that as perfect accuracy, or 1. The denominator P(S is tested positive for the D) is a bit more complicated. P(S is tested positive for the D) is the probability that S is tested positive for the disease and there are two ways that this could happen. Firstly, S might actually have the disease and has tested positive for it. Since we know 1 in 1,000 people have D and the test is perfectly accurate, we put down 0.001 x 1. Secondly, S might be among the vast majority of people who do not have D but is tested positive because of the 5% false-positive rate of the test. For this possibility, we write 0.999 x 0.05. Since there are two (logically exclusive) possible ways for S to be tested positive for D, we add together the two values and get 0.05095. Thus, 0.001 divided by 0.05095 is approximately 0.0196 or 1.96%.

The intuitive reason why the number appears so low is because the odds are overwhelming likely that S belongs to the cohort of people who do not have the disease (999 to 1 odds) and she was unlucky enough to receive a false positive. To put it vividly, select 1,000 people. Among them, we are told that only 1 would have the disease. Yet, if we test all of them for it, 50 of them would get a false positive. The odds of you actually having the disease after you have tested positive for it would be 1 in 51, which is about 2%. The test did raise the probability that you have the disease in light of your positive test. Prior to it, you had a 1 in 1,000, or 0.1%, chance that you have the disease. After the test, the probability increases to 2%. Still, given how rare the disease is, the odds that you have the disease are still remarkably low even with a positive test.

As we mentioned, although Bayes' Theorem is virtually synonymous with subjective probability, it is in fact agnostic with regard to how we interpret a probabilistic claim. It is applicable to both probabilities as measurements of subjective confidence and probabilities as, say, measurements of frequency or objective chances. Bayes wrote little on how he intended to interpret probabilities. Indeed, our example here uses initial assignments of probabilities such as the 1 in 1,000 rate or the 5% false positive that likely come from empirical observations of the frequency variety.

How does Bayes' Theorem help us address the early worry that subjective interpretation of probability is simply too loose to be of any useful clinical applications? One way the proponents of subjectivism have attempted to address this challenge is by suggesting that, as we update our subjective probabilities in light of new evidence, we will eventually converge to the same percentage.[7] Although we can start out with wildly diverse subjective degrees of confidence, repeated updating with principles like Bayes' Theorem will eventually nudge our probability assignments towards the same set of numbers. One can even think of the convergence as nature shaking our probabilities towards the way the world is. Proponents of subjectivism who believe in convergence, I suspect, tacitly believe that rationality, or the way the world is, would punish those who assign radically bizarre subjective probabilities. With enough time, we will all learn our lessons and converge to some sane spectrum.

Given the importance of convergence for the viability of subjective probability, it is distressing that no indisputable account of convergence has been developed. To be sure, many proponents have offered sketches, but basic problems remain. For example, how long will the convergence process take? Is there evidence that convergence will even occur after a significant series of revisions? Moreover, as we continue the revisions, we will need to help ourselves to other initial probabilities that are also subjective. For instance, after I have revised my probability of A in light of B, I might encounter new evidence C that will now guide my revision using Bayes' Theorem. To determine P(A/C), I will need to have a value for P(C), and this initial and unconditionalized probability is once again subjective. It is entirely possible that some of these new subjective probabilities can "pull" our revisions further apart. Why would we think that in this sea of subjectivity, we would somehow magically be blown by wind onto the same probabilistic island? Finally, as a matter of fundamental difficulty, it seems intuitively obvious that some assignments of confidence are irrational or even incorrect. A father who thinks there is a 99% chance that his son will react aversely to childhood vaccinations is being irrational or perhaps pathological. How are we to account for that in a subjectivist account of probability? If the father has done the right Bayesian updating using subjective initial probabilities, it seems that he has not made any mistakes in his reasoning. Yet, his worry does not match with any *real* danger in the world, and this is what makes it irrational. Given the theories' detachment from objective chances, subjective probability theories would have a hard time accounting from the father's failure to *assess* threats correctly.

5.5 Propensity Interpretation of Probability: Hidden Power Redux

While frequency theories interpret probability as brute reports of observed samples and subjectivism treats probability as reports of personal confidence, propensity interpretations take probability to be an objective feature of the world. In the case of quantum indeterminism, the idea that some things in the world behave in a chancy fashion seems well-founded. According to standard understanding of quantum mechanics, the decay of a radioactive material, for instance, is indeterministic. In other words, the laws of nature and initial conditions do not necessitate quantum outcomes. The best we can do is to describe the probability that a quantum event will take place. The chanciness of these events is an objective characteristic of (some parts of) the world. When we make a probability claim, we are saying something that is either objectively true or false.

Proponents of the propensity interpretation, however, do not wish to limit their view to just quantum phenomena. When a physician suggests to her patient that he has a 90% chance of responding positively to a drug treatment for his allergies, she describes some propensity of the patient, according to the view. It is not a mere report of brute observations of comparable samples, nor is it an expression of her subjective confidence. The 90% is a fact *about* the patient. One can think of these kinds of objective propensities as features of the world that ground, justify, or even explain frequency distributions and rational assignments of subjective confidence. An analogy that might elucidate this idea is to revisit the concept of a dispositional property that we saw earlier in Chapter 3. Solubility of a sugar cube is a property of the cube. It does not manifest itself until we place it in water. Yet, it is a property of the sugar cube and it is likely the physical result of microscopic structures of sugar crystals. Probabilistic propensities to behave in a certain way are similar to dispositional properties. And like a sugar cube dissolving in water, the probabilistic propensity of an object waits in coils and manifests itself when placed in the proper context. Perhaps the patient reports improvements with his allergies 9 out of 10 times when he takes the medication. The propensity of the patient to respond to the drug explains the frequency of his positive reports. Moreover, once we have identified the physical propensity of the patient to respond to the drug, we might consider aligning our subjective confidence in the therapeutic benefit of the drug for this patient with the propensity. Propensity, in this respect, is conceptually prior to both subjective probability and frequency distribution.

As intuitively attractive as the propensity interpretation appears, there are some formidable challenges to the view. For starters, it is not clear what exactly is an objective propensity in a deterministic world. For a coin, is there a propensity to land heads up 50% of the time? Suppose we know all the specific physical conditions of the coin, the force that flips it, air resistance, and so on—how is there any indeterministic propensity about whether it will land heads (or tails)? We can determine exactly which side it lands on. When we say that the coin has a 50% chance of landing heads up, we are reporting our ignorance and not some objective chanciness about the coin; specifically, we do not know all the relevant physical factors that determine the outcome of a coin flip.

For more complex systems such as human beings, the number of factors that affect our physiology is remarkably vast. In principle, however, if we know sufficient details of a person's physiology, we can make accurate predictions of how a person would respond to a drug, for instance. Unlike quantum systems, at the level of human physiology, we are deterministic; that is, the laws of nature and initial conditions determine what happens. If this is correct, probabilistic claims about physiological responses are just expressions of our ignorance. They are not claims about intrinsic propensities for the person to behave one way or another.

The introduction of propensities as a real feature of things in the world might not add much to our analysis of probability. Suppose we attempt to determine the propensity of a patient to respond to certain drug. How would we do that? We can conduct a series of trials to see how often the patient responds to the drug and extrapolate the results as the propensity of the patient. However, we could save ourselves the trouble by just identifying the trial results with probabilities (as frequency) without introducing any innate propensity. The result is equally informative and useful. The addition of probabilistic propensity as an objective property of a system is unnecessary from the point of view of analyzing the nature of probability. It is akin to saying a person who has blue eyes possesses some disposition to develop certain genes, and these genes lead to the phenotypical blue eyes. The "blue eye disposition" does no work that a genetic explanation doesn't already do.

Finally, Paul Humphreys (1985) put forth a devastating objection against a propensity interpretation of probability. In standard probability calculus, conditional probabilities are "directionally agnostic." For instance, with the appropriate probability values, I can derive P(A/B) using Bayes' Theorem. These values can also let me derive P(B/A). From the point of view of probability calculus, all we know is that two events are statistically correlated; there is no implication that causal dependencies exist or, if they do, whether they run in one direction or another. Suppose the probability that the patient recovers from a disease given he takes a certain drug is 90%. The propensity theory would interpret that conditional probability as the patient's having a 90% propensity to recover when he takes the drug.

Using Bayes' Theorem (and initial probabilities), we can also determine the "reversed" conditional probability of the patient's taking the drug given he recovers. Bayes' Theorem is indifferent to the direction of the conditionalization; whether it be P(A/B) or P(B/A), the theorem applies equally. Nevertheless, if we interpret the probability of the patient's ingesting the drug given he recovers in a similar propensity manner, we end up with a senseless claim that the propensity of the patient's taking the drug given he recovers is X%. It borders on incoherence to say that a patient has a propensity to take a drug given he recovers.

To put the point more broadly, propensity interpretations of probability appear to be sensitive to causal directions, while standard probability calculus including Bayes' Theorem is insensitive to them. In order to have a full theory of probabilities as propensities, we will need a new system of probability calculus that respects directionality. Not only is there no such system, it is not clear how one might revise formal probability calculus to include metaphysical directions. Like logic and mathematics, probability calculus such Bayes' Theorem are "topic neutral." They apply to apples, magical fairies, clouds, imaginary numbers, and pierogis regardless of whether they are "connected" causally, magically, or not at all. To "fix" Bayes' Theorem in order to be sensitive to the directions of causality is to violate its topic neutrality; e.g., Bayes' Theorem only works if A is caused by B. Reject topic neutrality at your own peril! The cost might prove far steeper than any promised gains.

5.6 Living in a World of Uncertainties About Uncertainties

We examined three attempts to understanding probabilistic claims: frequency distribution, subjective probability, and propensity interpretation. There are, of course, other theories in the literature. Yet, these three theories represent three basic ways we can understanding what probabilities mean. For frequency distribution, its proponents think of probabilities as straightforward reports of the proportions of observations. These reports contain minimal metaphysical assumptions about the world: what you see is what you get, so to speak. They do not require us to commit to whether the world is deterministic or indeterministic. They do not entail that there are any hidden probabilistic powers in the things observed such that the distributions are the powers' observable manifestations. From the point of view of empiricism, frequency distributions prove the friendliest.

Difficulties emerge for frequentists when one attempts to extrapolate from these reports to claims about things that we have not observed (e.g., claims about the future or generalizations that include unobserved samples). Extrapolations of this kind, so important in medical research, require plausible solutions to Hume's problem of induction in addition to Goodman's gruebleen paradox. Here lies a sharp dilemma: if frequency distributions remain nothing but reports of observations, they are largely unproblematic but they would be of little research and clinical use. If the distributions venture beyond what was observed and inductively infer valuable projections, then they would confront a host of problems that have plagued inductive logic.

Another way to remain metaphysically minimalistic when it comes to understanding probabilistic claims is to interpret them as measurements of subjective credence. The use of Bayes' Theorem, for instance, can be tremendously useful in helping us assess the significance of clinical tests and public health initiatives. The failure to grasp conditional probabilities (e.g., one's confidence in having a disease given a positive test) can lead to widely inappropriate diagnoses and treatment plans. In this respect, subjective probabilities are immediately applicable without solving the problems attached to inductive logic. One of the ways subjective probability manages to avoid metaphysical problems about the *real* probability of an event is to offer a great deal of leeway in the assignments of subjective probabilities. Two individuals who disagree about the subjective probabilities of an event are both equally "correct." After all, these numbers merely reflect their personal degrees of confidence, and what is risky to one might be tolerable to the other.

Without some way to control for the assignments of subjective probabilities, however, subjectivists face the problem of applicability. A physician tells a patient that he has an 85% chance of surviving for five years is reporting her personal confidence. If there are no right or wrong assignments, how is the patient supposed to interpret that information?[8] To be of any use other than as reports of personal confidence, subjectivists must offer some way to adjudicate intersubjective disagreements of probabilities. One solution is to argue that our probabilities assignments, however divergent they might be at the start, will converge to some same spectrum of values as we repeatedly revise them using Bayes' Theorem. Alas, there is no convincing argument that this is in fact the case. Furthermore, the use of Bayes' Theorem requires the reliance of some prior probabilities. How are we to justify the use of certain numbers? If we rely on distributions from clinical trials, for instance, we find ourselves confronting the exact same issues that frequentists face. If we instead use other subjective measurements of confidence, it becomes even less clear that individuals with radically different probabilities beliefs will be able to rationally resolve their differences.

Rather than treating probabilities with empiricist kid gloves, one might be tempted to embrace a metaphysically more robust understanding of probabilities. The propensity theorists see probabilities as real properties within events or things in the world. By ascribing probabilities as real properties in the world, proponents of this view can solve (at least in principle) the intersubjectivity problem. When two people disagree about probabilities, there is a fact of the matter as to who is right. Moreover, a propensity account can also provide an explanation as to why we encounter the frequency distributions that we do. The reason why "3" comes up about one-sixth of the time is that the die *really* has the property of coming up "3" one-sixth of the time. No wonder that as we accumulate more rolls, we find that the ratio of "3"s in relations to all rolls approaches one-sixth.

Like the positing of any unobservables, propensity theorists have to defend how we can determine that an event or thing in the world really has the property in question. Indeed, for deterministic phenomena like the rolling of a die, it is difficult to say that a die has a propensity to come up "3" one-sixth of the time. If we know sufficiently many physical properties of the die such as its geometry, its weight, and the velocity of the roll, there is no uncertainty about which side will come up. The "chanciness" of a die seems to be nothing but a measurement of our ignorance. Moreover, even if we ignore all the metaphysical problems with the ascription of propensities, traditional probability calculus that includes Bayes' Theorem does not respect many of the intuitions of the propensity account. Propensities, as Humphreys notes, seem to be directional: a die when rolled has a propensity to come up "3" one-sixth of the time, but it coming up one-sixth of the time for "3" does not have a propensity that it be rolled. In order for the propensity account to be remotely plausible, we need to find some way to square propensity's metaphysically rich account with standard probability calculus that contains scantly any assumptions about causal directions and so on.

The problems we examined with these three accounts are indicative of the fundamental challenges to their respective approaches. Both frequency distributions and subjective theories treat probabilities as not real features of the world. As a result, trying to squeeze any projectability or normativity (correctness of a probability assignment) becomes a tall task. Propensity accounts, on the other hand, take probabilities to be real properties in the world. But, without a way of determining these properties, this approach appears to offer nothing more than what frequency theories already do. Most basically, when it comes to what we intuitively think of probabilities and what we want to do with them, accounts that are devoid of metaphysical assumptions like frequency distributions might be too thin, and accounts that are metaphysically rich like propensity might be too thick. Unfortunately, the ideal space between these two ends proves to be all too elusive.

Given the centrality of probabilistic claims in clinical and research medicine, it is imperative that we understand what probabilistic claims mean. Even if we assume that probabilistic claims are heterogeneous (that is, they consist of a variety of different types of claims with perhaps some expressing confidence and some frequency distributions), we still confront the daunting problems that each approach faces. Until some of these philosophical problems are solved, it might be wise of us to maintain a level of conservativeness in our interpretations and applications of probabilistic claims. The intimate connections among probability, explanations, and evidence suggest that the lack of clarity in the first might bleed into the latter two as well. Since evidential reasoning is not the only method of forming beliefs, we might explore other methods, such as prudential reasoning as advocated by American Pragmatists.[9]

Notes

1 We will discuss the justification for this answer later on in this chapter.

2 I once had a student who suggested that one had a 50% chance of contracting HIV. Alarmed by her assessment, I asked for evidence. She replied, "Well, either you have it or you don't. So, it is 50–50."

3 The details of his argument can be found in Book 1, Part iii, and Section 6 of *A Treatise of Human Nature* (1738) and Section iv of *An Inquiry Concerning Human Understanding* (1748).

4 Alan Hájek argues that the reference class problem applies to other interpretations of probability as well. See his brilliant and wonderfully titled paper "The Reference Class Problem is Your Problem Too" (2007).

5 One of the most common definitions of what constitutes a coherent probability assignment is to rely on the concept of a Dutch Book wager. A Dutch Book wager is one in which no matter how events unfold, the bettor will always lose money. For instance, suppose I offer you a pair of bets. For outcome A, I offer you 9 to 10 odds and your bet price is $90. For outcome B, I offer you 1 to 4 odds and your bet price is $20. You must place both bets and only one outcome will occur. If A occurs, you would receive a $100 but you would have also paid $110 for both bets. If B occurs, you would receive $100 but you would have also paid $110. Regardless of what the outcome is, you would lose $10. We can identify the axioms (for example, the probability of any event must be greater than or equal to 0, the sum of the probability of A and the probability of not-A is equal to 1, etc.) by determining the minimal set of constraints that an assignment of probabilities must satisfy in order to avoid Dutch Books.

6 One can see an immediate contrast between subjective interpretation of probability and variations of the Principle of Indifference. Some theorists have suggested that the best way to understand Laplace's theory is to see it as an epistemic guideline. When one faces a series of options (that are jointly logically exhaustive) and one has no *reason* to believe that one outcome is more likely than another, one *should* assign all outcomes with the same probability. Radical subjectivism flaunts this normative recommendation. There is no requirement that one assign identical probabilities to subjectively indifferent choices so long as one satisfies the basic axioms of probability.

7 Hawthorne (1994), in a rather technical paper, provides three models of how subjectivists can rely on Bayes' Theorem to continuously update their probabilities and converge to the same confidence level. Convergence via repeated probability updating thus offers intersubjective agreements while relying on radically subjective initial assignments of probabilities.

8 A friend once relayed an experience in an emergency room that I think is particularly telling. Her physician suggested that the standard protocol was to keep her overnight for observation. My friend asked what the physician would do if she was in my friend's situation. The doctor replied that she would probably go home. This example nicely captures the subjectivity of probability and how we can use them interpersonally. Assume

that you have my prior probabilities: what do you think my conditional probability is? Surrogate decision-making or even advice-giving may very well be probabilistic empathy: pretend that you have my probability assignments, what would you do?

9 See James (2014) for a classic defense and articulation of prudential reasoning.

References

Casscells, W., Schoenberger, A., & Graboys, T. B. (1978). Interpretation by physicians of clinical laboratory results. *New England Journal of Medicine*, *299*(18), 999–1001. doi:10.1056/nejm197811022991808

Hájek, A. (2007). The reference class problem is your problem too. *Synthese*, *156*(3), 563–585.

Hawthorne, J. (1994). On the nature of bayesian convergence. *PSA: Proceedings of the Biennial Meeting of the Philosophy of Science Association*, *1994*, 241–249.

Hume, D. (2000). *A treatise of human nature*. Oxford, UK: Oxford University Press.

Hume, D. (2008). *An enquiry concerning human understanding*. Oxford, UK: Oxford University Press.

Humphreys, P. (1985). Why propensities cannot be probabilities. *The Philosophical Review*, *94*(4), 557–570. doi:10.2307/2185246

James, W. (2014). The will to believe. In W. James (Ed.), *The will to believe: And other essays in popular philosophy* (pp. 1–31). Cambridge: Cambridge University Press.

Laplace, P. S. (1852) [1812]. *A philosophical essay on probabilities*. New York, NY: Dover Publications.

Manrai, A. K., Bhatia, G., Strymish, J., Kohane, I. S., & Jain, S. H (2014). Medicine's uncomfortable relationship with math: Calculating positive predictive value. *JAMA Internal Medicine*, *174*(6), 991–993. doi:10.1001/jamainternmed.2014.1059

6

VALUE-FREE MEDICINE

6.1 Care Without Values?

In providing medical care, clinicians are taught not to impose their personal values in diagnostic and therapeutic interactions with their patients. The idea that the patient's input has as much, if not more, weight in determining their therapeutic path is a relatively recent phenomenon. Often referred to as the "shared decision-making" model of the physician-patient relationship, the idea is that clinicians work together with patients to identify their treatment plans. In this partnership, clinicians interpret and present relevant medical information while the patients decide what they want.

A half a century earlier, however, patients hardly had a voice in determining their care. Physicians diagnosed and recommended treatment; patients listened and accepted their advice like children being told what was best for them. Female patients and those from vulnerable populations (e.g., racial minorities) were often afforded even less respect for their preferences. Lawrence Henderson (1935)—a physician, philosopher, and sociologist who served as the director of Harvard Medical School—writes:

> In your relations with your patients you will inevitably do much harm, and this will be by no means confined to your strictly medical blunders. It will arise also from what you say and what you fail to say. But try to do as little harm as possible, not only in treatment with drugs, or with the knife, but also in treatment with words, with the expression of your sentiments and emotions. Try at all times to act upon the patient so as to modify his sentiments to his own advantage, and remember that, to this end, nothing is more effective than arousing in him the belief that you are concerned whole-heartedly and exclusively for *his* welfare.
>
> *(823)*

Although it is clear that Henderson's intentions are noble, this sort of extreme paternalism presupposes that physicians know their patients' interests (or "advantage" in his words). It might seem obvious to most care-providers that a patient wants to continue to live with a reasonable level of quality of life. But this assumption comes from the clinicians' values, and it might not be shared by their patients.

Oncology presents some of the clearest examples of how values play an important role in therapeutic decision-making. For a given type of cancer, there are often numerous protocols to treat it. These protocols differ in terms of outcomes and treatment experiences. For instance, one protocol might maximize a patient's long-term prospects at the expense of greater toxicity during the treatment; another might trade survival for better post-treatment quality of life. And, of course, forgoing any treatment in favor of supportive care is also a viable alternative for some patients.[1] Without knowing a patient's values, it would be wholly inappropriate to recommend one protocol over another. A clinician cannot simply assume that every patient shares her preferences.[2 3]

Henderson's piece was published in the 1930s. Some might dismiss it as a relic of a less-enlightened era of clinical medicine. But we continue to find examples of advocacy for paternalism in the second half of the 20th century. Bernard Meyer, clinical professor of psychology at Mt. Sinai School of Medicine, wrote in 1969:

> [W]hat is imparted to a patient about his illness should be planned with the same care and executed with the same skill that are demanded by any potentially therapeutic measure. Like the transfusion of blood, the dispensing of certain information must be distinctly indicated; the amount given must be consonant with the needs of the recipient, and the type must be chosen with the view of avoiding untoward reactions.
>
> *(68)*

Since clinicians presumably are experts at the executions of treatments, if truth disclosure is akin to a blood transfusion, then clinicians and clinicians alone know what patients need to know.

We can view the shared decision-making model as a response to the paternalistic orthodoxy. Unlike radical paternalism, the shared decision-making model aims to ensure that clinicians do not impose their values on their patients. In the 2014 version of the American Counseling Association's *Code of Ethics*, under section A.4 entitled "Avoiding Harm and Imposing Values," the ACA urges that:

> Counselors are aware of—and avoid imposing—their own values, attitudes, beliefs, and behaviors. Counselors respect the diversity of clients, trainees, and research participants and seek training in areas in which they are at risk of imposing their values onto clients, especially when the counselor's values are inconsistent with the client's goals or are discriminatory in nature.
>
> *(ACA, 2014)*

This commitment to a value-free medicine, stemming from a recognition of the importance of patients' autonomy, extends beyond the physician-patient relationship. Hospital ethics committees are often discouraged from making ethical recommendations as solutions to the moral problems that they are tasked to assist, especially when there are multiple morally permissible courses of actions. The American Society for Bioethics and Humanities' *Core Competencies for Healthcare Ethics Consultation: The Report of the American Society for Bioethics and Humanities* (2011) recommends that:

> [C]onsultant should refrain from unduly influencing the patient's decision. . . . Ethics consultants need to be sensitive to their personal moral values and should take care not to impose their own values on other parties. This requires that consultants be able to identify and articulate their own views and develop self-awareness regarding how their views affect consultation.
> *(9)*

Although healthcare reimbursement and coverage policies (from insurance companies and government programs) occasionally hold patients responsible for their life-style choices (e.g., smokers pay higher insurance premiums), by-and-large, moral responsibilities do not come into play when we allocate medical resources. Whether one's injuries were the results of a skiing accident or falling down a flight of stairs, healthcare coverage rarely discriminates. Again, one of the main reasons is a general respect for diverse life-style choices: medicine does not want to be in the business of making judgments about what values are worthy of living by and worthy of care.

In light of our strong commitment to a value-free medicine, we ought to be clear about what values are and where they show up in clinical and research practices. Is it possible to have a value-free medicine? If so, is it something that we actually want? If not, how should we structure our practices so that they incorporate the value-laden nature of medicine? This chapter and the next one tackle these issues. We begin with an exploration of values in clinical medicine. In the next chapter, the discussions will center around the relationship between values and research medicine.

6.2 The Nature of Values

A helpful first step to understanding the nature of values is to contrast them with facts. Values typical include considerations like happiness, friendship, meaningfulness of one's chosen activities, morality, autonomy, and so on. These are things that are important to each of us. In general, philosophers see matters of facts and matters of values as mutually exclusive; matters of facts are capable of being true or false (sometimes referred to as "truth-apt") while matters of values are not. This quick-and-dirty distinction, however, is not entirely correct. Imperative statements like "Pass the salt" are neither true nor false. We surely do not want to say that they are matters of values. One might try instead to define what a value is by suggesting that if something is valuable, then one ought to bring about more of it. This is also incorrect. Humans are valuable in that they have some intrinsic worth (e.g., they have rights and so on). It would be bizarre to say that because people are valuable, we should create more people.

We might be tempted to say that facts are objective and values are subjective. But, again, we run into trouble when we are pressed to say more about the objective/subjective distinction. If by "subjective," one means it concerns a particular agent and not other people, then a patient's MRI is subjective. Surely, this is not what we mean by subjective. If we instead say that something is subjective if it makes references to an individual's preference, it is certainly a fact that the individual has that preference. But what makes that preference itself not factual? Is it because it is not truth-apt? If so, we are back to square one with our analysis of the truth-value distinction.

Indeed, the concept of value likely consists of a number of different subgroups.[4] We will not attempt to give a comprehensive account of all varieties of values. We will focus rather on the concepts of values that are germane to the practice of clinical and research medicine. For this chapter, specifically, we will look at the types of values that are relevant to clinical medicine: concepts such as patients' values, values in diagnostic and therapeutic decision-making, value impositions by clinicians and institutions, and so on. These are considerations that guide a person's actions. For instance, if I place a value on my ability to play the piano, one can infer that, all else being equal, I would safeguard and nurture my ability to play the piano. Similarly, if a physician values patients' privacy, it entails that, all else being equal, she would choose the course of action that maximizes the protection of that privacy.

The connection between values and actions is arguably a distinguishing characteristic between matters of value and matters of facts. It is a factual judgment that the Earth is largely spherical, but the acceptance of this fact alone does not guide our actions, per se. Contrast it with the claim that lying is wrong. If we accept this claim, then there is a prima facie prescription for our actions; perhaps something like, all else being equal, one *ought* not to lie. Philosophers often refer to this quality as the normative nature of values; that is, matters of values set up norms for actions—they tell us how we ought to act. Value claims are thus often referred to as "ought-claims" and factual claims as "is-claims."

There is no doubt that values play significant roles in how we live at a global-level and a local-level. The fact that one values intellectual pursuits might lead one to choose educational and career paths that maximize these activities. More locally, one might choose to go to a restaurant that is family-friendly because one might place a value premium on being able to eat with one's family. Given the ubiquitous nature of values, it is a bit surprising that science has historically eschewed values and strived to cleanse its pursuit to be free of them.

One argument in favor of this approach perhaps began with David Hume's well-known "is-ought gap." In Book III of *A Treatise of Human Nature* (1738/2000), Hume writes:

> In every system of morality, which I have hitherto met with, I have always remarked, that the author proceeds for some time in the ordinary way of reasoning, and establishes the being of a God, or makes observations concerning human affairs; when of a sudden I am surprised to find, that instead of the usual copulations of propositions, is, and is not, I meet with no proposition that is not connected with an ought, or an ought not. This change is imperceptible; but is, however, of the last consequence. For as this ought, or ought not, expresses some new relation or affirmation, it is necessary that it should be observed and explained; and at the same time that a reason should be given, for what seems altogether inconceivable, how this new relation can be a deduction from others, which are entirely different from it. But as authors do not commonly use this precaution, I shall presume to recommend it to the readers; and am persuaded, that this small attention would subvert all the vulgar systems of morality, and let us see, that the distinction of vice and virtue is not founded merely on the relations of objects, nor is perceived by reason.
>
> *(Part I, Section I)*

Hume is arguing that attempts to derive value claims from factual claims always leave an argumentative gap unfilled. It is not laziness that is responsible for the missing step; rather, his point is that no ought-claim can be derived solely from is-claims. Philosophers refer to this conceptual gap as the "is-ought gap."

Take this argument that seeks to establish the moral impermissibility of euthanasia.

(1) Euthanasia involves the deliberate killing of a person.
Therefore, euthanasia is wrong.

As it stands, the argument is invalid; after all, there are many acts of deliberate killing that do not strike us as morally wrong, such as self-defense or capital punishment. In order to make the argument valid, we need to add a new premise such as (2) The deliberate killing of a person is wrong. This premise, however, contains the value term "wrong," and we no longer have a set of purely factual premises. Hume proposes that no amount of non-value premises alone can ever entail a value conclusion.

The Cambridge philosopher G.E. Moore noted 165 years later a similar fissure between what is the case and what ought to be the case. In his *Principia Ethica* (1903), Moore argues that the "naturalistic" definition (defined using non-moral terms) of moral concepts will always fall short. Take the concept "good." A classic hedonistic utilitarian might define "good" as that which maximizes happiness for the most people. Moore claims that although the statement "good is good" is trivially true, "good is that which maximizes happiness for the most people" is certainly not. We can always ask *why* that which maximizes happiness for the most people is in fact good. Moral terms (and values for our purposes) are ultimately indefinable in terms of non-moral or naturalistic terms. Indeed, Moore suggests that moral terms behave much like color terms like "yellow": we can know all its naturalistic qualities (e.g., its typical wavelengths), but it would be a mistake to define yellow as just these qualities. Philosophers have labeled Moore's argument as the "Naturalistic Fallacy" or the "Open-Question Argument."[5]

One of the most well-known responses to Moore (and Hume) is called Cornell Realism. It is so called because the main proponents all developed their views while they were at Cornell as faculty or students. Borrowing from how we understand scientific concepts, the philosopher Richard Boyd (1995) argues that a moral concept like "goodness" behaves a lot like "healthiness." Just as being healthy is not directly observable, being good is a concept that we infer. We can identify observable and naturalistic factors that contribute to a person's health (e.g., blood pressure and skin tone) and, noticing these factors, can make informed judgments about the relative healthiness of a person. A healthy person can also exhibit health by behavior—she is more likely to be able to do things that she desires, her life is likely longer, and so on. Boyd suggests that we understand moral concepts like goodness analogously. First, we identify the functional role goodness plays, and we locate the "upstream" factors that affect moral goodness and the "downstream" factors that goodness can affect. An action causing pain, for instance, might play an upstream role in that we are more inclined to conclude that an act is wrong if it causes pain. Moral goodness can have downstream effects as well, in that it might lead to, say, a greater chance of human flourishing or peace. Drawing conclusions about morality on the basis of observable facts presents no greater challenge, in principle, than understanding concepts like "healthiness."

Criticisms and defense of Cornell Realism have generated a great deal of debate within metaethics. A fundamental problem with Cornell Realism is that, like healthiness, identifying the naturalistic factors that causally contribute to it (and are causally affected by it) is no simple matter. As we noted in Chapter 2, figuring out just which physiological factors are relevant to the concept of healthiness seems to depend on certain value assumptions. Declining eyesight as one ages, though annoying, is not considered unhealthy because we think it is normal not to be able to see as well with age. What is normal is of course dependent on norms and values. Boyd's project assumes that we have some ways to identify the relevant causal factors that affect the goodness of something. Is the fact that a public policy makes many people unhappy a contributing factor to it being bad? Moore's naturalistic fallacy precisely points out the impossibility of answering that question.

Here we see the beginning of medicine's commitment to being value-free. If values are non-factive (i.e., they are neither true nor false), to impose one set of values on someone who doesn't share them is to impose something that cannot be rationally justified by facts alone. Perhaps it is in this sense that we think of values as subjective: they reflect our personal preferences much like one's favorite ice cream flavor. It would be contrary to our respect for a patient's autonomy for a clinician to impose her values on her patients. Just because she likes rocky road ice cream, it doesn't follow that she has grounds to insist that her patients also like rocky road ice cream. To be sure, we often limit someone's autonomy or try to change the person's mind. When I see that you are boarding a train to New Haven after you have told me you wish to travel to New York City, I might pull you off the train paternalistically. I can defend my intervention on the grounds that your action was inconsistent with your expressed desire to go to New York City and that you were literally wrong about what train you were boarding. However, to insist that you actually want to go to New York City instead of New Haven is to impose my values onto you, and there is, according to Hume and Moore, no factual reason to defend that. Limiting someone's autonomy as such would be rationally groundless or philosophically arbitrary, one might say.[6]

6.3 The Collapse of the Fact-Value Distinction

Philosophers have long acknowledged the difficulties in delineating a clear distinction between facts and values. Consider an example from the philosopher Hilary Putnam (2002) of a concept that seems to straddle the distinction: cruelty. A historian might consider Emperor Nero a cruel individual. Is this a factual claim or a value claim? To determine whether historically Nero was cruel, we might look to factual records of his heinous acts and edicts. If the rumor proves true that he started the Great Fire of Rome in 64 CE just so that he could rebuild it as he saw fit, this historical fact certainly lends credence to the claim that Nero was cruel. At the same time, to call Nero cruel is to make certain moral claims. A cruel act is something that one *ought* not to do; cruelty appears to entail behavioral prescriptions—a hallmark of value terms. Putnam suggests that there is much vagueness between facts and values. A sharp distinction between the two is either unwarranted or artificially created.

The blurring of the distinction between facts and values in analytic philosophy in the past 50 or so years has largely gone asymmetrically; that is, philosophers have realized that a concept of facts that treat them as value-free is exceedingly difficult to defend. What causes the collapse of the fact-value distinction is that there appear to be no value-free facts or value-free ways of learning about them. One of the most dramatic ways we can appreciate the centrality of values in rational pursuits is to recognize their presence in the most basic of human reasoning—logic.

In classical logic, one can derive a sentence "P" by showing that an assumption of "not-P" leads to a contradiction. This inferential strategy is often referred to as *reductio ad absurdum*, or reduction to absurdity, and it has been a handy logical move since the Ancient Greeks. Around the start of the 20th century, logicians and mathematicians such as L.E.J. Brouwer questioned whether inference rules such as *reductio* are in fact legitimate. Their objections stem not from any logical critique per se; they are not concerned with whether the rule ensures that if the premises were true, the conclusion must be true (that is, validity) in classical logic. Rather, the issue is whether from a philosophical point of view one is entitled to draw a conclusion for something without an actual positive proof for it. In the case of a *reductio* argument for "P," one is not actually constructing a proof for "P"; instead, one is proving that the denial of "P" leads to a contradiction. There is no independent proof for "P," so to speak. Being more conservative with what constitutes legitimate rules of reasoning, Brouwer and other logicians developed entire systems of logic that reject some of the rules of classical logic, including *reductio*. The resulting systems are known as intuitionistic logic or, because of the desire to have an independent positive proof for each conclusion, constructivist logic. Their writings on the matter, amazingly, often involve as many technical details as they do grand and mystical musings on the nature of rationality. Because of their rejection of the rules of classical logic, intuitionistic systems are less powerful in that they can prove fewer theorems.

Suppose we ask the big question: who is right? The answer depends heavily on one's personal philosophies about what is important.[7] For instance, Brouwer was motivated by his (unorthodox) belief that logical proofs are "mental constructs." When one decides whether or not to adopt intuitionistic logic, one must ask whether its lesser inferential power can be justified by the benefits of being consistent with some antecedent philosophical views. For Brouwer, he was willing to pay the price of adopting a less powerful logic because it squared with his metaphysical beliefs about logical proofs being mental constructs. Philosophical cost-benefit analyses of this sort require us to assess the relative weight of the two conflicting desiderata. What is more *valuable* to us: adopting a logic that is consistent with our other philosophical views, or having the ability to prove more things? Our answer must consider not only pragmatic values such as convenience; it also often includes epistemic factors such as certainty, tolerance of the risk of being wrong (e.g., how certain are you that your metaphysical beliefs are true?), and the cognitive cost of rejecting other beliefs in order to accommodate the adoption of a system of logic. These factors surely contain personal values.

If choice of logic is value-laden, then every inferential move, all of rationality, and all the conclusions we draw will be "tainted" by certain value-judgments. We infer facts, confirm them, reason using them, and act upon them. All of these would require logical reasoning, the adoption of which, as we saw, contains values. Whether the conclusions we draw are logically justified would thus turn on matters of values.

Once we move beyond the realm of deductive reasoning and consider inductive or abductive reasoning, the presence of values becomes even clearer. Take inference to the best explanation. What constitutes "enough" evidential support (for us to believe a hypothesis) is determined by values (one might, for instance, trade certainty in exchange for expediency because one thinks life is too short: we cannot wait forever for "sufficient" evidence to come in). Similarly, weighing the relative importance of criteria like simplicity, applicability, degree of empirical adequacy, elegance, fruitfulness, computability, etc. are all dependent on individuals' values. The collapse of a sharp distinction between facts and values is the result of our growing recognition that there are no conclusions we can draw rationally without assuming some values.[8]

6.4 How We Live with Values

Hume's and Moore's arguments have sparked a tremendous amount of philosophical discussion not only in ethics but also in the philosophy of science. Indeed, one can appreciate the efforts of the early positivists to purge philosophy of value claims by following Hume's recommendation that anything that is neither conceptual nor empirical should be committed to the flames.

Our discussion of science vs. pseudo-science in Chapter 1, especially Thomas Kuhn's work, also demonstrates the challenges values pose to the traditional view that science is in the business of discovering objective facts about the world. It is no coincidence that the emerging recognition of the centrality of values in modern science has been accompanied by a deflation of the grand view of science as a truth-seeking enterprise. One can even think of Evidence-Based Medicine as an attempt to bring more objectivity into clinical care, and that values (being unchecked by truths and falsities) present an incompatible influence on medicine. If we are to be more objective, the argument goes, we need to eliminate as much personal preference as possible. EBM is thus the inevitable result of two assumptions: medicine should be value-free and medicine guided by EBM is (fairly?) value-free. As we recognize the importance of protecting patients from unwanted value impositions, we look for more ways to practice medicine without value assumptions. EBM represents the ultimate solution: the impersonal ways of science will now ensure that personal biases from clinicians cannot enter therapeutic recommendations.

Most philosophers today recognize that Hume and Moore were right about a great many things regarding values. The idea that one can simply jump from what *is* naturally the case (as defined factually) to what *ought* to be the case will almost instantaneously solicit cries of "naturalistic fallacy!" For example, to conclude that genetic modifications are wrong because they are not done naturally (e.g., they cannot be done without artificial interventions) is to make precisely the kind of mistake that Hume charges. Nevertheless, many philosophers also tend to be skeptical of the alleged unbridgeable chasm between is-claims and ought-claims. The American philosopher Judith Jarvis Thomson, for example, articulates her suspicion nicely:

> An act's being an instance of "causes a person pain" is not conclusive proof that it is wrongful, for surely it could be, and in some cases is, permissible to cause pain (as, for example, where the victim will die if not caused pain

> and prefers pain to death). But that fact about an act is certainly favorably relevant to its being wrong.
>
> *(1990, p. 15)*

In determining the wrongness of an act, finding out that it causes pain increases the plausibility that the act is wrong. Thomson's idea here echoes Boyd's "upstream" concept we mentioned earlier. Perhaps Hume and Moore are right that we cannot *deductively* derive moral claims on the basis of factual claims alone. But there are non-deductive modes of reasoning, from inference to the best explanations to pragmatism.

In a series of three lectures originally given in 2007 as the annual Tanner Lectures on Human Values at Princeton University, the American philosopher Susan Wolf (2010) alludes to our implicit belief that not all values are created equal. Wolf's broader project concerns the question of what makes a life meaningful. One popular response that she examines is the recommendation that one should live doing what one loves. Here Wolf points out that, however plausible the view can be, some choices simply strike us as less meaningful. She writes:

> Not all actions that are motivated and guided by reasons of love are justified, however. Not all reasons of love are good reasons. . . . [L]ove can be misplaced or misguided; the energy and attention that you give to an object may be disproportionate to what that object merits. A wonderful woman might give up her career, her home, her friendships to follow and serve a man the rest of us see clearly does not "deserve her". An impressionable teenager might sign over his trust fund to a cult with which he has become enamored, thereby losing both his financial security and the opportunity to benefit worthier and needier groups.
>
> *(6)*

Just because one wants to do something, it doesn't follow that it is something one *ought* to want. Identifying those values that are worth having from those that are not is by no means an easy task. Wolf points out an obvious critique of this type of objectivity in the value of values. She refers to it with the self-explanatory name "who's to say." For medicine, subscribing to the objectivity of values clearly exposes us to the threat of elites or those who are in power (e.g., clinicians) to dismiss patients' values and substitute them for their own "enlightened" ones. Wolf is cognizant of the dangers and the challenges of explicating what activities are objectively valuable and, alas, she does not provide definitive solutions.

The great 19th century British philosopher, co-founder of utilitarianism, and economist John Stuart Mill argues persuasively for a kind of liberalism that tolerates life-style choices that one would not condone (1999). His argument for tolerance essentially draws from our inability to rationally adjudicate the relative merits of competing values. And, in the name of avoiding errors and imposing ungrounded conclusions, one must tolerate seemingly valueless life-choices. It is

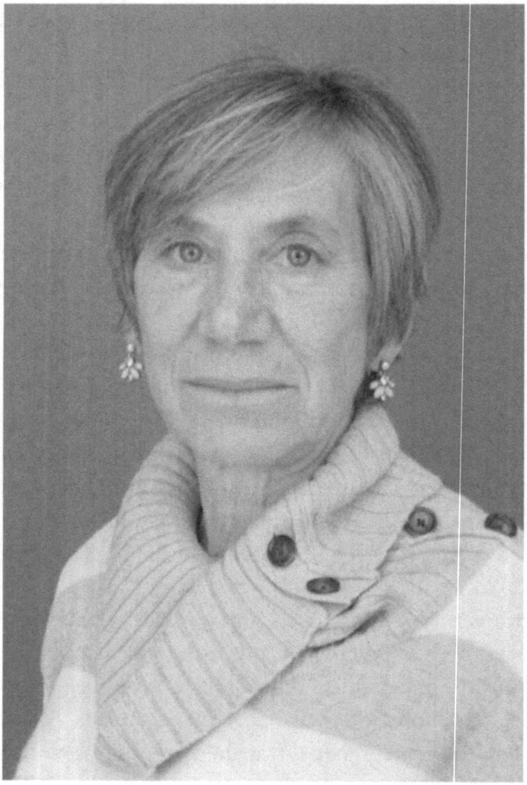

FIGURE 6.1 Susan Wolf

Susan Wolf has eloquently suggested that meaning arises when "subjective attraction meets objective attractiveness." *Source:* Image courtesy of Susan Wolf and UNC-Chapel Hill.

important to note that even for the defender of classic liberalism, Mill, like Wolf, saw the alleged superiority of some values over others; it is our inability to justify the ranking that leads to radical tolerance. Unlike his fellow utilitarian founder Jeremy Bentham, Mill advocates for a preference of higher over lower pleasures (where the former correspond to intellectual pursuits—a rather convenient delineation for an academic). In his *Utilitarianism* (1863, p. 14), Mill famously writes that "[i]t is better to be a human being dissatisfied than a pig satisfied; better to be Socrates dissatisfied than a fool satisfied." The question, it appears, is not whether we think sad Socrates lived a better life than a happy fool, but how we can identify and justify these alleged differences.

A goal of normative ethics is to account for how and why ethical agents like ourselves behave the ways that we do. Acting as if values are not all equal is certainly one of our more salient moral behaviors. Clinicians do not always follow or maximize a patient's articulated values. Just because one would like titanium

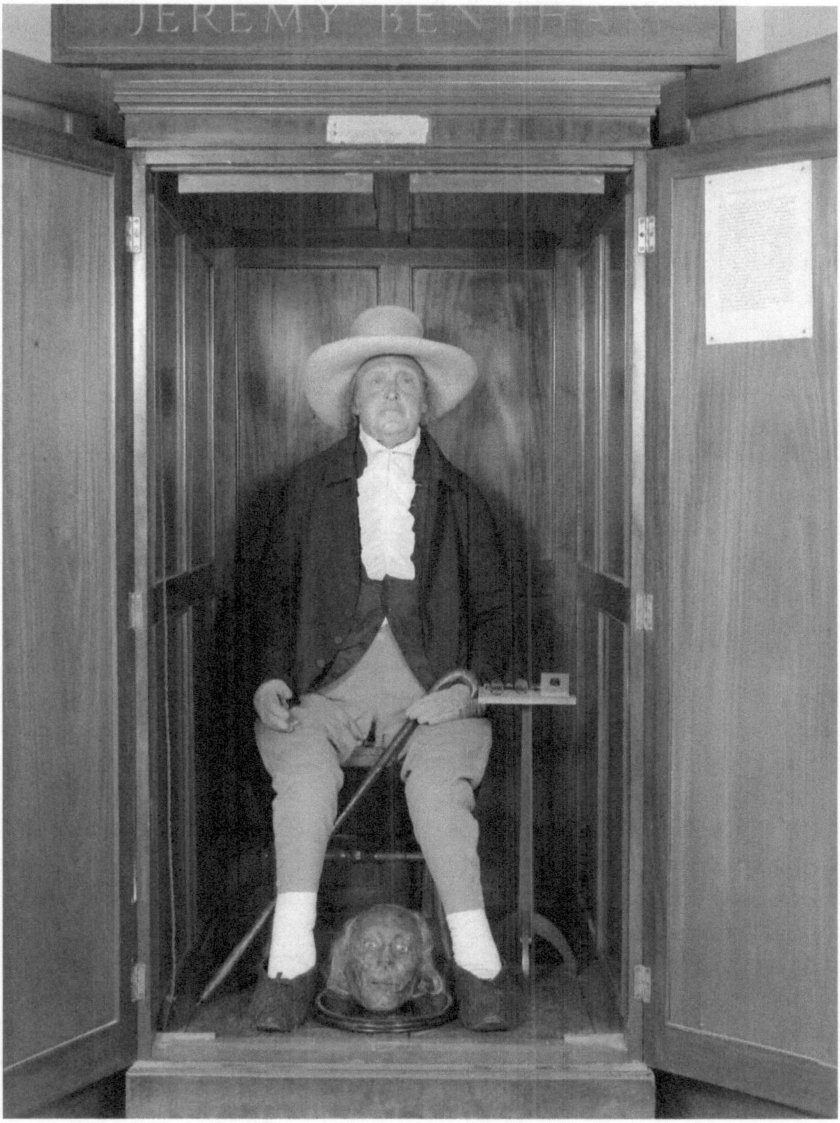

FIGURE 6.2 Jeremy Bentham

Jeremy Bentham's preserved and donated body is displayed at University College of London. Between his feet lies Bentham's actual head which, due to poor preservation techniques, had to be replaced by a wax replica. The irony of a utilitarian who thought of pleasures as the guiding elements for how one ought to live is not to be missed. After all, directives after death bring no pleasures to the deceased, and perhaps even displeasure for those in the company of the auto-icon. *Source:* © UCL Galton Collection, UCL Culture.

whiskers implanted into one's lips and just because the desire is incredibly strong, most physicians would at least hesitate to perform the surgery. The reluctance goes beyond the lack of medical necessity (for physicians occasionally provide medically unnecessary interventions), nor is it merely a matter of the patient's safety (for physicians do provide elective and potentially risky services). The suspicion is that making one look like a cat is not the sort of thing that most physicians find worthy of value. Whether this is right or wrong is a separate issue. The relevance here is that if ethics is about capturing our salient ethical judgments or behaviors, it would be *prima facie* inappropriate for us to ignore our common practice of treating the merits of values as being objectively varied.

6.5 Can Medicine Be Value-Free?

The shared decision-making model of the physician-patient relationship departs from the traditional paternalistic model by taking seriously patients' values in the determination of their therapeutic directions. The model is ambiguous, however, in terms of the role patients' values play. How determinative should they be? How much should a clinician respect them? Ezekiel Emanuel and Linda Emanuel (1992) identify four models of the physician-patient relationship starting from the paternalistic model that respects patients' autonomy the least to the informative model where physicians keep their hands off patients' values (Table 6.1).

Consider the "informative model." Within this relationship, they argue that physicians do not shape or even elucidate patients' values. Their role is to provide patients with plain medical facts about the benefits and challenges of various treatment plans. The patients then take this information and make up their minds about what best maximizes their values.

Though seemingly living up to the cliché "just the facts, ma'am," the informative model already presupposes certain values from the physicians' point of view. In articulating medical information, clinicians must decide the level of detail, the inclusion of plausible and relevant treatment, and patients' degrees of comprehension. Even the most educated patient who is very familiar with the physiological aspects of her condition will likely not know all the pertinent information. A clinician who presents a treatment plan must edit down and interpret medical information. These choices require the clinician to know something about what qualifies as a good enough amount of detail for the patient to act upon. Moreover, she must also judge when the patient has understood it well enough. These are both normative choices physicians make on behalf of their patients.

In addition to depth, there is also the width of medical information a clinician must consider when choosing to communicate available treatments. Perhaps she has read an experimental study out at a distant clinic that has shown some promise, but she thinks it is far too risky and costly for her patient to consider it. Should she disclose it because it is, after all, *a* possible treatment plan? Furthermore, clinicians also do not disclose treatments that have been replaced by newer

TABLE 6.1 Emanuel and Emanuel's four models of physician-patient relationship

	Informative	*Interpretive*	*Deliberative*	*Paternalistic*
Patient's values	Defined, fixed, and known to the patient	Inchoate and conflicting, requiring elucidation	Open to development and revision through moral discussion	Objective and shared by physician and patient
Physician's obligation	Providing relevant factual information and implementing patient's selected intervention	Elucidating and interpreting relevant patient values as well as informing the patient and implementing the patient's selected intervention	Articulating and persuading the patient of the most admirable values as well as informing the patient and implementing the patient's selected intervention	Promoting the patient's well-being independent of the patient's current preferences
Conception of patient's autonomy	Choice of, and control over, medical care	Self-understanding relevant to medical care	Moral self-development relevant to medical care	Assenting to objective values
Conception of physician's role	Competent technical expert	Counselor or adviser	Friend or teacher	Guardian

approaches. If there are more effective drugs available with fewer side-effects, it makes little sense for anyone to choose a drug that is apparently inferior. But this assumption is a value assumption that clinicians make on behalf of their patients. Even for "standard" therapeutic recommendations, we can see how they contain implicit value assumptions. After oral surgeries, clinicians often recommend a round of prophylactic antibiotics to lower the patient's risk of infection. The use of antibiotics is not without cost both to the patient and the general population. It is entirely possible that a patient desires to accept the higher risk of an infection because he feels strongly that the marginal benefits of prophylactic antibiotics do not outweigh the contribution they make to the acceleration of the emergence of antibiotic-resistant pathogens. His decision is clearly based on personal values. In medicine, as in life, what is wise for one person might be foolish for another.

The ubiquitous presence of values even in the most mundane elements of clinical medicine raises some doubts about whether there can be such a thing as value-free medicine. Indeed, communications and social interactions invariably require us to make decisions that are driven by value assumptions. A friend once relayed a story about American GIs overseas. On a particularly hot day, a group of them were about to cool off in a body of water. One GI asked a local, "Are there crocodiles in the lake?" The local replied, "No." As the GIs jumped into the water, a crocodile started to snap its jaw, chasing the band out of the water. "I thought you said there were no crocodiles in the lake!" one complained. The local replied, "That's a river. Not a lake."

In semantics, it is a widely accepted theory that information we convey to one another depends on shared social values and contexts. Much of the information is not explicitly stated but rather comes from conversational implicatures. When one asks if there is a gas station nearby, the context makes clear that one is looking for an open gas station. It would be a cruel joke to send the inquirer to a gas station that one knows has been closed for years. Medicine as a social and communicative practice must contain values, some of which are not trivial. When proponents of value-free medicine advocate for the avoidance of personal values, they surely do not mean that medicine should contain absolutely no values whatsoever: communication, at least, would be tremendously cumbersome, if not impossible. What they mean, instead, is that some value assumptions are permissible and some are not. The question for us is not whether medicine should be value-free, but which values we should adopt in the practice of medicine.

6.6 The Consequences of a Value-Laden Medicine

Recall that the fear of a value-laden clinical medicine rests primarily on medicine's respect of patients' autonomy. There is of course an obvious way to reconcile the presence of values in medicine with the premium we place on patients' autonomy: why not just ask patients what their values are and act upon them? If we let patients' values guide their clinical interactions and therapeutic decisions, the probability of a patient's autonomy being compromised is slim.[9] There are two problems with this reply. Firstly we assume that patients know what their values are and that they can communicate them to their clinicians. Even the most reflective (and healthy) individuals can have a difficult time articulating what they care deeply about. Moreover, our values are often inconsistent: one might value living a life that maximizes what one enjoys while recognizing the importance of one's less-than-pleasant financial duty to take care of family members. When these values conflict, their resolutions are far from clear; indeed, they are arguably the basis of much of our existential angst. In addition, given the limited interactions most patients have with their clinicians (partly due to cost-containment pressure from insurers), it seems unlikely that patients can engage in the type of meaningful conversations that can elucidate and share their values. Secondly, even if we can overcome these technical problems, we still need to consider the limits of respecting patients' values. As we discussed in the last section, we certainly behave as if not all values are equally worthy of our respect. Indeed, medical conscientious clauses exist in part to allow clinicians to decline requested services that they deem unreasonable or unsavory. An absolute respect of patients' values is neither realistic nor defensible.

As Wolf has conceded, we have no accepted way of arguing why some values are not worthy of equal respect. Even if we agree that value progress (or "changes," if one were to use a less loaded term) is possible, it is not clear if we know the "logic" of how we should revise our values. We have no principle that can tell us that, given a certain value P, in light of new information Q, how one should revise P. For instance, for someone who loves veal and cares about animal welfare, finding out that the production of veal causes a great deal of distress should at least nudge that individual away from his love of veal. Yet, there is no Bayesian updating for values, so to speak.

An objective prioritization of values is difficult, if not impossible to define. But the fact that we often change our ethical views in light of new information (be it factual or not) gives us hope that there is a way to accommodate values in medicine without violating patients' autonomy. The key is to recognize that although values cannot be checked by logical consistency the same way that beliefs can, there is still a sense in which values can hang coherently or incoherently together. It is this appeal to coherence that will give us some tools to engage each other in value-discourse. We can change each other's mind, critically reflect on our own choices, and, relevantly, practice medicine in a way that respects autonomy and recognizes its value-laden nature.

6.7 The Web of Values

In earlier chapters, we discussed Kuhn's concept of a scientific paradigm, which consists of an inter-related system of beliefs within which the "important" ones occupy a central core and the less important ones the peripheral. When an observation conflicts with our paradigm, we restore logical consistency by revising our peripheral beliefs. Adjusting the outer beliefs causes the least amount of disruption to our paradigm. This kind of coherentism predates Kuhn's views, and it is not only limited to the philosophy of science. The American analytic philosopher W.V.O. Quine is well-known for his more basic version of epistemic coherentism, or holism.[10] Quine's idea is that our epistemic views of the world consist of a web of beliefs (like Kuhn's paradigm later): core beliefs such as arithmetic and logical truths are those upon which most of the peripheral beliefs depend. When an observation impinges on the web, we revise our beliefs with a principle of conservation; we make the necessary revisions to restore logical consistency that requires the least amount of disruption to our web.

One of the most controversial results of Quine's view is that there is nothing in principle that prohibits us from rejecting any belief, including core ones, if we are willing to pay the massive cognitive price of a radical revision. Indeed, a Quinean might look to the rejection of core classical logic principles in light of bizarre experimental results in quantum mechanics as an example of the dictum "nothing is sacred."

In the case of beliefs, it is easy to see how consistency demands the reconciliation of logically incompatible ones. When holding the belief P and ~P, we can restore consistency by rejecting at least one of them. The case for values, on the other hand, is more complicated. Unlike beliefs which can be either true or false, values might not be truth-apt as we understand them. If I value both P and ~P, the inconsistency by definition cannot be a matter of logic; that is, I am holding a set of beliefs that are both true and not true. Someone who has contradictory values is not being logically inconsistent. We all have our nuisances when it comes to matters of taste. We can at once recognize that a movie is simply awful and still enjoy it as a "guilty pleasure." One might even proclaim that one *ought* not to like this movie but still find it irresistible. It is peculiar and curious (perhaps it might even reveal some interesting psychological facts about us), but it is not illogical in any strong sense.

Without truth, how are we to articulate the apparent inconsistencies in our web of values? Consider the recent debate in the United States on the legalization of same-sex marriage. Some opponents of legalization argued that same-sex marriage should not be sanctioned on the grounds that the intended purpose of marriage is to procreate. Same-sex couples lack (unassisted) means to do so; therefore, they should not be allowed to be married. A powerful reply is to point out that states recognize the right of infertile couples and of couples who do not wish to have children to be legally married. If we permit marriages in the case of non-child-bearing heterosexual couples, consistency requires that we ought to accept the right of same-sex couples to be married as well. At the very least, the inability of same-sex couples to procreate without artificial intervention is not sufficient reason to deny them their right to be married. Other attempts to distinguish same-sex marriages from heterosexual marriages also failed along similar lines. The force of these replies, I surmise, swayed public opinion enough that poll after poll showed an increased willingness to legalize same-sex marriage across the country.

The most important lesson to learn from these real-life cases of practical reasoning is that we often use them in public discourse, convince one another, and make progress in our disagreements. We might not have a thorough account of the metaphysics of moral claims, but we behave as if values can be checked by reasons. Obviously, it is possible that proponents of the non-rationality of morality and values are right and that we have been fundamentally wrong that morality can be guided by reasons. But, the burden of proof—and a burdensome one it is—rests on those who wish to convince us that morality is not what it seems. At the very least, to jump to the practical conclusion that values have no role to play in medicine because there is nothing right or wrong about values is too quick.[11] There are many legitimate reasons why one might wish to minimize the role of values in medicine. Nonetheless, the reason cannot be the strong metaethical claim that values cannot be properly guided by reasons. To do so is to adopt a philosophical position when the jury is still very much out.

Given the apparent unavoidability of values in medicine, our strongly held belief that values can be checked by reasons, and our implicit commitment that not all values are equal (e.g., Wolf's view), insisting on a value-free medicine is likely unwarranted. Practical reasoning techniques such as arguments by parity give us some tools to resolve value disagreements. Of course, we might still wonder why we wish to have "consistent" values. The answer to this question not only justifies our ideal of value consistency, it also can tell us a great deal about the limits of our tolerance for inconsistencies. Surely, in a liberal democracy, one does not *have* to be completely consistent in one's values in order to enjoy a level of respect as an autonomous agent. At the same time, we also believe that not all inconsistencies of values are to be tolerated. We allow physicians to refuse to treat on conscientious grounds, but we do not allow physicians to refuse treatment because they do not like their patients' races. Just because differing values are respected, it doesn't follow that one can hide one's bigotry behind metaethical debates. In public life, we have a plethora of mechanisms to settle social disagreements, from direct democratic referendum to townhall outreach, that ensure all stakeholders are heard and their values considered. The end result might not be right, but it will be fair.

6.8 How Medicine Can Learn From Life

We began this chapter asking whether value-free medicine is possible, and if it is, whether it is good to pursue it. Our discussion leads us to the conclusion that values invariably exist in medicine; thus, the real question is which value we should tolerate and how. One of the central arguments for value-free medicine is the non-factive nature of values: they do not seem to be the sort of things that can be either true or false. This realization has led many to conclude that any appeal to values (perhaps other than the patients') will degenerate into non-rational value impositions that threaten patients' autonomy. Given the premium we place on the latter, at the very least, values should play as small of a role as possible.

As we saw, from Hume's is-ought gap to Moore's naturalistic fallacy, there are plenty of reasons to worry that values cannot be appropriately guided by reasons. Nevertheless, our ordinary beliefs and practices show that we strongly believe otherwise. To eschew values in medicine on metaethical ground is, I argue, philosophically premature. Given the availability of practical reasoning tools that we use outside of medicine to resolve value disagreements, it is unwarranted to give up on values entirely in clinical medicine. They are not as unmanageable and dangerous as many think; just look at how you live and maneuver in the real world, steeped in competing values.

In addition to the philosophical reasons why many reject values in medicine, there are also non-philosophical or quasi-philosophical ones. From a historical and political point of view, appealing to favored values has been the trademark of some of the greatest abuses and exploitations both in medical history and social history. Forced sterilization performed by doctors in Nazi Germany or advanced by eugenic policies in the U.S. had a veneer of paternalism: many victims were sterilized for their own good. These practices speak to the horror of letting values run amok, and our admirable desire to maintain a value-free medicine is a safeguard to ensure that these abuses do not happen again. Likewise, one might argue that since we have no way of determining some objective ranking of the worthiness of values to be respected, we should adopt a cautionary approach and lean on the side of minimizing values in medicine.

In response to these legitimate concerns, we should keep in mind the fact that values do exist in medicine. Rather than ignoring their presence, we might be better off recognizing them and borrowing tools that we have in ordinary life to tackle them. A value-free medicine is not harm-free. As most clinicians have noticed, patients' requests for exoteric and often expensive treatments have been increasingly met by clinicians who tread gingerly, not wanting to impose their values on the patients. Some clinicians' willingness to do as asked comes from clinicians' growing habit of practicing defensive medicine.[12] Some of it, I suspect, comes from the prominence of patients' autonomy in clinical ethics. Just as we manage to live and to strive in other social relationships when matters of values arise (even when the stakes are high), it is not improper for us to structure a clinical medicine that openly recognizes the importance of the values of all parties involved. In the next chapter, we will look at Helen Longino's proposal that science ought to embrace its value-laden nature and decide proactively what kind of values it should be guided by. Her recommendations for research medicine may prove helpful to clinical care as well.

Notes

1 Quill (1991) writes about his experience with a 45-year-old cancer patient who declined treatment. Quill's initial difficulty understanding the wish of a patient to forgo a 25% chance of survival eventually gave way to his support of her desire to seek assistance from the Hemlock Society to end her life. His change of attitude stemmed from long conversations with his patient during which he learned of her values.

2 Learning about a patient's values is not just a matter of ethical medicine. If a goal of medicine is to restore the autonomy a patient lost to diseases and disabilities, then knowing a patient's values is indispensable in a clinician's recommendation of the most suitable treatments.

3 There are some subtle philosophical distinctions that are being glossed over. Preferences and values might not be the same thing, for instance. Intuitively, I believe being a vegetarian is a value I hold. I also enjoy eating chocolate, but it would be odd to say that eating chocolate is a value. Some of these issues will hopefully be cleared up as we say a bit more about the nature of values. However, some of them will be left vague for the sake of scope.

4 The concept "good," for example, can show up in a wide variety of usages. A good chess move, a good person, a good deed, a good movie, and so on might contain different meanings of "good." There might be a fact of the matter that a chess move is good, when there is none when it comes to the goodness of a movie. For a more detail discussion, see Chapter 1 of Ridge (2014).

5 Moore offers another argument that challenges the coherence of analyses in general. For instance, it is trivially true that water is water, but not so for water is H_2O. If "water" just *is* "H_2O," then surely we should be able to substitute one for the other without any changes in the truth or the meaning of sentences containing them. Known as "The Paradox of Analysis," to disarm this argument, one needs to deploy some rather sophisticated theories of semantics and so on. It is worthwhile to distinguish Moore's Naturalistic Fallacy from his Paradox of Analysis. In the case of the former, Moore's claim can be understood as about the plausibility of defining a moral concept in terms of non-moral ones. This interpretation echoes Hume's argument. In fact, the similarity between the two have led some to refer to Hume's argument as the naturalistic fallacy as well.

6 Indeed, we can draw a similar conclusion without even making the assumption that matters of values are neither true nor false (a metaphysical claim). All we have to assume is some skepticism towards our ability to identify the objectively correct values (an epistemic claim). To wit: if we have no means of justifying the correctness of some values, then it would be prima facie inappropriate for me to impose them onto you.

7 The diversity of logical systems includes not just classical logic and intuitionistic logic; there are also other non-classical systems (often referred to as deviant logic) that offer different degrees of inferential power. Paraconsistent logic, for instance, typically rejects classical logic's acceptance that one can derive anything from a contradiction. Similarly, some systems of tri-valued logic introduce "undetermined" as an addition to the classical values true and false. There are also systems such as supervaluationist logic, fuzzy logic (where any real number between 0 and 1 can represent a truth value), quantum logic, and so on. Whether there is a "true" system of logic is certainly an open debate in philosophy. As things stand, different logical systems are often treated as tools for different tasks. The choice is more a matter of pragmatic determination than any robust claim that there is an objectively correct system.

8 There is obviously a difference between there being no purely value-free facts and there being no value-free ways for us to identify these facts. The former is a metaphysical claim about whether value-free facts exist, and the latter is an epistemic claim about whether we can identify them without assuming some values. Confusing metaphysics with epistemology is a great sin among philosophers. Nevertheless, from the point of view of applied practices like clinical and research medicine, not being able to derive conclusions without assuming values is just as bad as there being no value-free facts. American Pragmatists are fond of saying that the quest for justified beliefs (epistemic) and the quest for truth (metaphysical) look indistinguishable. For clinicians and researchers, it matters little whether value-free facts exist. A value-free medicine is doomed if we cannot epistemically identify facts without assuming certain values.

9 We are taking a rather simplistic view that respecting patients' preferences and values is both necessary and sufficient to safeguard patients' autonomy. This is a complex matter. If one believes that autonomy is defined on the basis of acting as a fully-informed rational agent, then a patient's explicitly stated values and preferences might have no bearing on her "real" autonomy (if she is not fully informed, say). The objectivity of values might come into play as well. A patient might say she values X but she might be wrong—X is not the sort of things that is valuable.

10 Quine wrote numerous publications on the topic of epistemic holism. The classic is *Two Dogmas of Empiricism* (1951), in which he launches some of his strongest critiques against logical empiricism championed by his teacher Rudolf Carnap. His positive thesis is a recommendation to embrace some form of epistemic holism.

11 The claim "we *ought* not to include values in medicine" runs the risk of self-refutation.

12 In a fascinating study, Sakoulas, Wormser, Visintainer, Aronow, and Nadelman (2009) identify a positive correlation between the rate of unnecessary prescriptions of antibiotics and concentration of attorneys. They suggest that doctors are prescribing more antibiotics in these areas because they fear potential litigation.

References

American Counselling Association (ACA). (2014). *Code of Ethics*. https://www.counseling.org/knowledge-center/ethics#2014code. Accessed 3/30/2019.

ASBH. (2011). *ASBH core competencies for health care ethics consultation*. Glenview, IL: American Society for Bioethics and Humanities.

Boyd, Richard N. (1995). 15 How to be a moral realist. In Paul K. Moser & J. D. Trout (Eds.), *Contemporary materialism: A reader* (p. 297). Abingdon: Routledge.

Emanuel, E. J., & Emanuel, L. L. (1992). Four models of the physician-patient relationship. *JAMA, 267*(16), 2221–2226.

Henderson, L. J. (1935). Physician and patient as a social system. *New England Journal of Medicine, 212*(18), 819–823. doi:10.1056/nejm193505022121803

Hume, D. (2000). *A treatise of human nature*. Oxford, UK: Oxford University Press.

Meyer, B. C. (1969). Truth and the physician. *Bulletin of the New York Academy of Medicine, 45*(1), 59–71.

Mill, J. S. (1999). *On liberty* (Vol. 55). Peterborough: Broadview Press.

Mill, J. S. (1863). *Utilitarianism*. London: Parker, Son, and Borne.

Moore, G. E. (1903). *Principia ethica* (Vol. 13). Mineola, NY: Dover Publications.

Putnam, H. (2002). *The collapse of the fact/value dichotomy and other essays*. Cambridge, MA: Harvard University Press.

Quill, T. E. (1991). Death and dignity. *New England Journal of Medicine, 324*(10), 691–694. doi:10.1056/nejm199103073241010

Quine, W.V. O. (1951). Two dogmas of empiricism. *Philosophical Review, 60*(1), 20–43.

Ridge, M. (2014). *Impassioned belief*. Oxford: Oxford University Press.

Sakoulas, G., Wormser, G. P., Visintainer, P., Aronow, W. S., & Nadelman, R. B. (2009). Relationship between population density of attorneys and prevalence of methicillin-resistant staphylococcus aureus: Is medical-legal pressure on physicians a driving force behind the development of antibiotic resistance? *American Journal of Therapeutics, 16*(5).

Thomson, J. J. (1990). *The realm of rights*. Cambridge, MA: Harvard University Press.

Wolf, S., Koethe, J., Adams, R. M., Arpaly, N., Haidt, J., & Macedo, S. (2010). *Meaning in life and why it matters*. Princeton, NJ: Princeton University Press.

7

TRUTH AND HAPPINESS

7.1 The Crumpling of the Great Firewall

The syphilis studies at Tuskegee, the hepatitis trials at Willowbrook, and the demonological experiments done by Albert Kligman (a co-developer of Retin-A) on prisoners at Holmesburg Prison in Philadelphia are three of the better-known unethical experiments done on human subjects in the United States. The fact that they took place after World War II (Tuskegee started in 1932 but did not end until 1972), after the horrors of unethical human experiments were brought to light by the discovery of the Nazi experiments, made them all the more disturbing. We had developed the Nuremberg Code to safeguard human subjects in response to the atrocities of those Nazi experiments. We were the good guys in the war. We couldn't and wouldn't do what they did. Yet, the most cursory look at the history of medical research in the 20th century shows American hands have not been clean.

It seems remarkably easy to pinpoint exactly why these experiments were unethical. Vulnerable children at Willowbrook State School, who often had serious developmental challenges, were given chocolate milk deliberately tainted with feces from children with hepatitis. Performing experiments on children that do not benefit them raises significant moral challenges, even with parental consent. Revelations that parents were told their children could only be admitted to Willowbrook if they consented to participating in the experiments only made it more difficult to justify what was done to this vulnerable population.[1]

Horrific experiments like this are often assumed to come from morally unscrupulous researchers. Their greed, bigotry, and biases lead them to disregard ethical safeguards and the worth of their subjects. Although biographers and historians can tell us if this was true, the implicit belief is that science is morally neutral: it is how and what we do with science that is affected by our values and biases. Science can tell us if our theories of thermal-nuclear explosion are supported by evidence, but science cannot tell us whether we *ought* to build a hydrogen bomb. This great firewall between the inner workings of science and the personal values of the scientist was a major tenet of the positivist movement. Indeed, the hope was that once we discovered the "logic of science," we could ensure that science is conducted independently of subjective biases. Logic and evidence supplied by nature would be the ultimate arbiters of scientific disagreements. Regardless of whether you are good or evil, science can judge the merit of your work qua science.

The second half of the 20th century saw the crumbling of the great firewall. We have slowly realized that the inner workings of science are hardly as clean and objective as the positivists had thought. Worse still, philosophers such as Helen Longino and Kathleen Okruhlik have argued that external values can covertly enter our "logic" of science. Researchers' biases and values can affect what constitutes good science. As we will see, science is a deeply value-laden practice that reflects our beliefs of what is important. For those who appreciate the fact that science is done by real people with human frailties (rather than abstract algorithms for hypothesis-selection), this might not come as a surprise. However, the value-laden nature of science is not just a matter of sociology and psychology; it is a matter of philosophy. The value-laden quality of science is a consequence of limitations and particularities of how we understand the world around us. In other words, science is value-laden because we cannot understand the world without using values.

To use Helen Longino's terminology, we make a distinction between constitutive values and contextual values. Longino explains:

> I distinguish two kinds of values relevant to the sciences. Constitutive values, internal to the sciences, are the source of the rules determining what constitutes acceptable scientific practice or scientific method. The personal, social and cultural values, those group or individual preferences about what ought to be I call contextual values, to indicate that they belong to the social and cultural context in which science is done (Longino, 1983). The traditional interpretation of the value-freedom of modern natural science amounts to a claim that its constitutive and contextual features are clearly distinct from and independent of one another, that contextual values play no role in the inner workings of scientific inquiry, in reasoning and observation.
>
> *(1987, p. 54)*

The claim that constitutive values shape how we reason within science is uncontroversial, given the ubiquity of values in theoretical reasoning. The more significant claim is that, according to Longino, contextual values (those that structure the institutional and social aspects of science) can also affect scientific reasoning (the inner workings of scientific inquiry, as she puts it).[2]

We will end the chapter with a broad exploration of how we should understand medicine if values become unavoidable. It is both a moral and political imperative that we are mindful of these hidden agents. At the very least, we should recognize that they exist and that they affect the way we practice medicine. In light of this conclusion, perhaps we must choose what kind of values we want in medicine—these choices are partly dictated by what we ultimately want from clinical and research medicine. Our discussion in Chapter 1 of the goals of medicine will come full circle in this final chapter.

7.2 Constitutive Values in Medicine: Values Within Scientific Reasoning

Theoretical or scientific reasoning clearly involves values, although the extent to which values guide the inferences we make is up for debate. There are at least three main areas where values play significant roles:

(1) The formal and informal algorithms we use to make inferences in science;
(2) The characterizations of observations; and
(3) The inferential gap between evidence and the hypotheses one seeks to support (the problem of underdetermination).

In Longino's terminology, constitutive values affect the "inner" workings of scientific reasoning—they make up the workings of science. Throughout the course of the first five chapters, we have encountered numerous instances where values guide scientific reasoning. Let us take an inventory and make some broad observations about how and why values are unavoidable in scientific reasoning.

For the first category, values are entrenched in the formal and informal algorithms we use to reason in science. As we saw in the last chapter, which system of deductive logic we choose depends on our broader philosophical commitments and personal values. It might be rational for someone to adopt classical logic over intuitionistic logic, even if she believes that the latter is more compatible with her metaphysical beliefs. The uncertainty of the truth of her metaphysical beliefs, for instance, might give her enough pause to adopt classical logic. She would rather adopt a system that can let her prove more theorems than one that is weaker but is compatible with her metaphysical views—she values inferential power over her metaphysical beliefs. Alternatively, she might use classical logic because the profession at large uses it, and she would rather avoid the hassle of adopting an esoteric system. Since logic underlies most, if not all, of our principles of reasoning (scientific or formal), the choices we make here on the basis of personal values mean that every logical inference we accept flows from the same well of values.

More concretely, the choice of setting statistical significance at $p = 0.05$ is obviously a matter of value. We can adopt a higher statistical standard (as many scholars have advocated) and thereby lower the risk of false-positives. The trade-off between certainty and sustainability of scientific research is a matter of priorities. We deem that it is simply not worth the price of making studies prohibitively expensive to run by insisting on a lower *p*-value for the benefits of greater certainty. Likewise, the convention we choose for the number of digits sufficient for scientific significance is also determined by values. One might argue that insisting on more than n significant digits is a waste of resources because ordinary (read: affordable) measuring devices in question cannot reach a greater-than-n degree of precision. Of course, whether it is a waste or not is a matter of values and, similarly, whether uncertainties and possible errors are worth tolerating is also a matter of values.[3]

When it comes to inductive reasoning, the role of values become even more obvious. In Chapter 3, we discussed Goodman's solution to the new problem of induction. To wit, the basic problem is that we cannot distinguish regularities that are genuine laws from those that are not. Although we might think "green" can participate in a law (i.e., it is projectable) and "grue" not, we do not have a way to justify the different treatments. Since whether a piece of evidence supports a hypothesis depends on the projectability of the terms, unless we can sort projectable terms from non-projectable ones, we do not know what hypothesis can afford confirmation by evidence.

Goodman suggests that what makes a predicate projectable is merely that it has been entrenched: we started building our scientific worldview around it. There is nothing in principle that distinguishes projectable and non-projectable predicates. If Goodman is correct, our reluctance to accept "grue" (or, more relevantly, "intersessional prayers for better health") as projectable ultimately rests on our unwillingness to shake up our worldview too much. The values we place on stability over time, avoidance of radical changes in our worldview for very little benefit, and good old laziness guide our decisions.

In the case of abductive reasoning or inference to the best explanation, values also determine inferential support. A plausibility of a hypothesis, according to IBE, depends on its ability to explain the evidence. In the legal system, jurors are instructed to reach a verdict beyond a reasonable doubt; that is, they identify the hypothesis—guilt or innocence—that best explains the evidence presented. When they conclude that the defendant is most likely guilty of the alleged crime, they are not required to consider and dismiss *all* or even *most* doubts. Such a system of jurisprudence would be unworkable, though it would lessen the chances of convicting an innocent person. We decide that the benefit of having a relatively speedy system of justice is worth the price of accepting some level of uncertainty and some conviction errors. An analogous trade-off takes place in scientific reasoning: we can always have a lower *p*-value, we can always control for more confounders, and we can always run a clinical trial longer. We choose not to do these things because the value we place on a "good enough" research science that gives us practical applications is greater than whatever epistemic gains we could otherwise achieve.

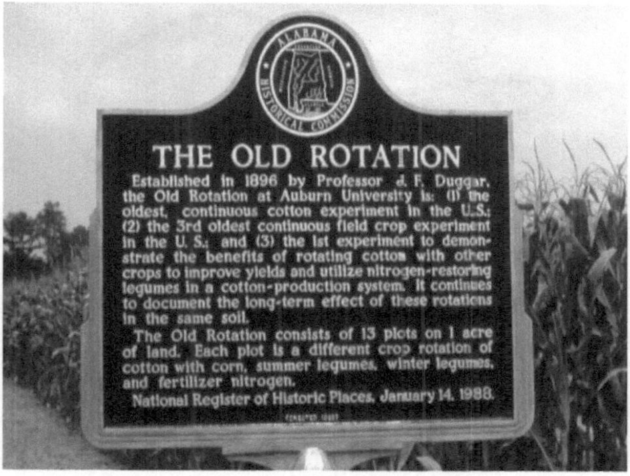
ALABAMA
HISTORICAL COMMISSION
THE OLD ROTATION
Established in 1896 by Professor J. F. Duggar, the Old Rotation at Auburn University is: (1) the oldest, continuous cotton experiment in the U.S.; (2) the 3rd oldest continuous field crop experiment in the U. S.; and (3) the 1st experiment to demonstrate the benefits of rotating cotton with other crops to improve yields and utilize nitrogen-restoring legumes in a cotton-production system. It continues to document the long-term effect of these rotations in the same soil.
The Old Rotation consists of 13 plots on 1 acre of land. Each plot is a different crop rotation of cotton with corn, summer legumes, winter legumes, and fertilizer nitrogen.
National Register of Historic Places, January 14, 1988.

FIGURE 7.1 Old Rotation

The Old Rotation at Auburn University started as an experiment to determine if soil could support cotton growth indefinitely if crops of legume were rotated in during winter months. The experiment started in 1896 and continues today. Presumably, the conclusion enjoys a tremendously low p-value. *Source:* The original uploader was Saverivers at English Wikipedia., https://commons.wikimedia.org/wiki/File:TheOldRotation1.JPG, "TheOldRotation1," https://creativecommons.org/licenses/by-sa/2.5/legalcode.

The second area where values pop up in the inner workings of science comes from the philosophical idea that observations are always theory-laden. The traditional (e.g., positivist's) theory of observation is that observations present "raw" data from the world with which we can adjudicate the relative merits of competing hypotheses and refine and develop accepted ones. However much a scientist might wish her theory squares with reality, the traditional view tells us that nature is impartial and it supplies objective data that adjudicate scientific disagreements.

The Cambridge philosopher Ludwig Wittgenstein notes in his celebrated *Philosophical Investigations* (1953) that observations do not come pre-sorted. Observers often see the world in a kind of "seeing-as." To illustrate his point, Wittgenstein offers a classic ambiguous image—the duck-rabbit.

For Wittgenstein, an observer can view it *as* a duck or *as* a rabbit. There is no objective fact of the matter whether it is in fact a duck or a rabbit. Philosophers like Thomas Kuhn, Paul Feyerabend, and Norwood Hanson argue that the phenomenon of "seeing-as" extends beyond ambiguous images but to all observations. In other words, observations are not "clean" reports; instead, they are always couched in the theoretical language of the observer such that any observation reports presuppose the acceptance of some theories on the part of the observer.

A basic medical in medical imaging can help illustrate the point. Take a look at this venogram of the left subclavian 77-year-old man who needs a replacement

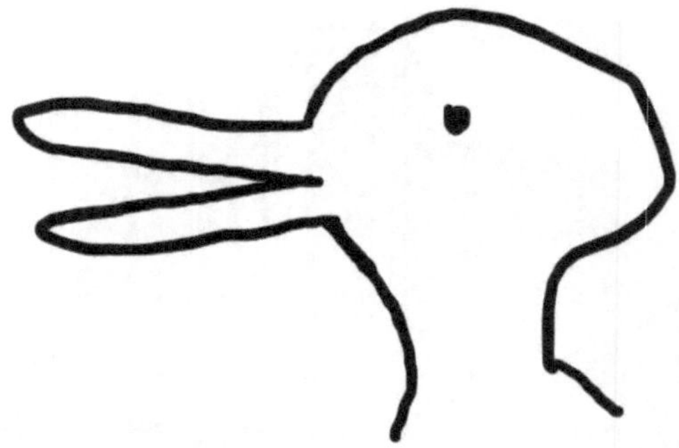

FIGURE 7.2 Duck-Rabbit

of his implantable cardioverter-defibrillators—a heart rate monitoring implant that would send electrical shocks to the heart if it detects dangerous irregularities.

With trained eyes, Magnusson and Kastberg (2017) diagnose a stenosis of the left subclavian vein (at the arrow point in Figure 7.3). What we see, as laypersons, is a bunch of gray squiggles with some thicker than others. To see the veins, the abnormal narrowing, and a lesion in the superior vena cava require training in not only physiology but also radiography. Without knowledge of these prior theories, one could not see these indicators of the ailment. The clinician sees the narrower gray squiggle *as* a high-grade stenosis.

The phenomenon of "seeing-as" is not unique to science. Exposure to training in art history allows one to see things in paintings that one would otherwise not notice. The texture of the paint, the reaction to a prior master, the play of space and solid, and a subtle commentary on the political intrigues around the artist's life are only observable if one is armed with the right conceptual lens. The diversity of interpretation that one can make using different lenses is a part of what is fascinating about literary and artist interpretations. Seeing the same piece from a different point of view reveals new observations that one could not see before. What is true for art is true for science: observations reside within a theoretical context.

The problem of specifying how observations can be untainted by theories became a significant problem for the positivists. After all, they relied on them as theory-neutral evidence to settle theoretical disagreements. If observations are always theory-laden, they cannot serve as an unbiased judge. The danger is that the theories we use to describe the observation already stack the deck in favor of that theory. Moreover, what one sees from one theoretical perspective might not be what another sees. How then are we to say who is right when they can't even agree on what they are looking at? The quest for clean theory-neutral observations led positivists to some radical ends. Rather than saying, "I see the heart rate of the patient falling" (as a clinician watches the digital display of a heart monitor), a positivist might say, "I notice a visual stimulation on the lower right side of my

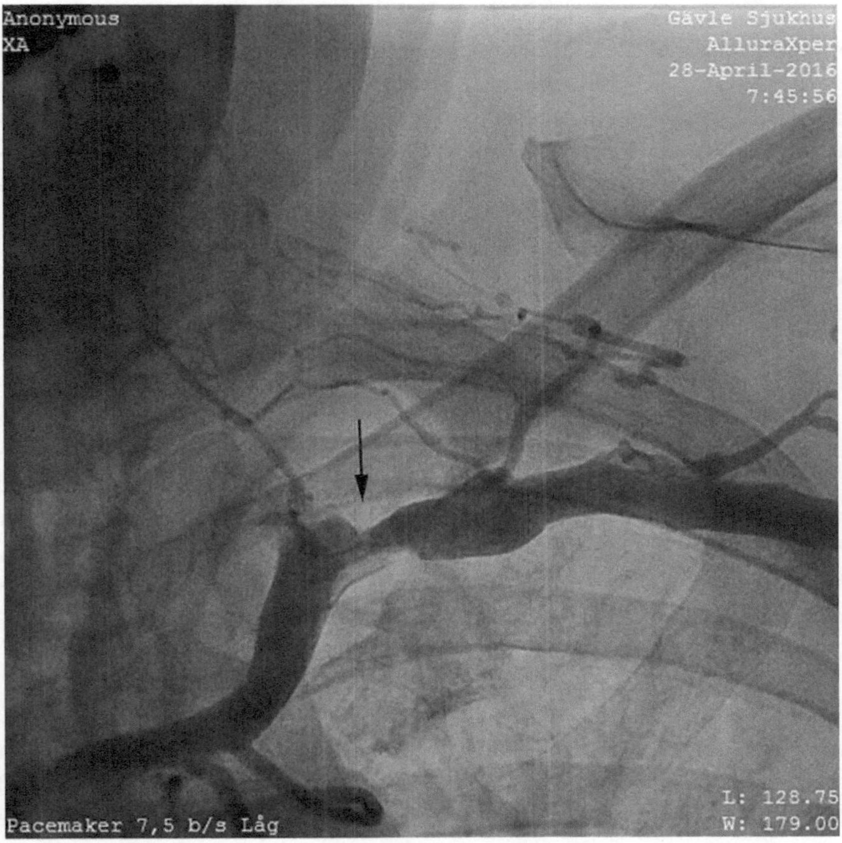

FIGURE 7.3 Left Subclavian Distal Stenosis

visual field. The stimulation resembles an arrow pointing downward while to its left are more flashing stimulations that appear like the number '42.'"

The problem with this attempt to couch observations in a hyper theory-neutral language is that science never makes reports or predictions of this sort. When Le Verrier predicted the existence of Neptune, his theory did not entail that when eventually observed, the planet would "stimulate the upper right area of the visual field with such-and-such intensity." Rather than a fine-grain prediction, his theory would tell us that when we have a powerful enough telescope, we would be able to see a planet on such-and-such a night. The raw-observation account fails because it construes scientific observations at a bizarre level of detail or in a manner that no actual scientific prediction makes. The fact that an astronomer pointed her telescope slightly off-center and ended up having a lower left visual stimulation did not mean that Le Verrier's theory was bunk!

Formal arguments for the theory-laden quality of observations by Kuhn and Feyerabend are more precise, but also more complex. One of the most well-known versions of the argument comes from Kuhn, and it is based on his view that the meanings of observation terms come from the theories within which they couch. Take the term "mass." As we recall from high school physics, classical mechanics tell us that inertial mass can be defined as F = ma. According to special relativity, however, there are two concepts of mass: rest mass, which is identical to Newton's concept, and relativistic mass, which constitutes a part of the measurement of energy within a system. The equation "$E = mc^2$" says that mass is in fact the amount of energy in a system divided by the square of the speed of light. While for Newton, mass is always conserved, relativistic mass is convertible to energy such that mass, by itself, is not conserved within a system. When an observer measures the mass of an object, what she means by "mass" depends on the theory from which the term "mass" comes.

Philosophers have hotly debated the extent to which the meaning of a term is defined by the entire theory surrounding it. In Kuhn's earlier writings, he suggests that two distinct theories have two distinct semantics (meanings for terms), and thus the two theories are in principle incommensurate. Kuhn's later comments, however, indicate that he might have walked back from this rather strong claim. For our purpose, we don't have to determine if Kuhn is right about the incommensurability of different theories. Instead, we only need to notice that the meaning of scientific terms draws from the theories that contain them.

Take the Chinese concept of "qi." Often translated as "life force" or "energy," a comprehension of the meaning of the term requires that one has a rudimentary understanding of Chinese theories of physiology. Qi flows through one's body via meridian paths. Key junctions, or meridian points, affect the functioning of vital organs, and ailments can arise when qi is flowing poorly. The use of acupuncture is one way to manipulate qi. Although the term literally means "air," the concept of qi in Chinese medicine comes with a robust theoretical background. Without understanding its role in this broader context, the meaning of qi would be lost to most. One standard way practitioners of Chinese medicine can detect qi is by placing their fingers on the inside wrist of a patient and feeling the pulse. When a practitioner notices that a patient's qi is weak, she makes an observation that non-practitioner could not "see." Kuhn's point is that all scientific concepts behave similarly. We see only what our theories let us see. Without theories, there are no observations.[4] Since the choice of theory is guided by values and all observations are theory-laden, it follows that all observations are dependent on certain values.

The third place where values can arise in research medicine is the perennial problem of underdetermination: a finite amount of observations can *never* single out a unique hypothesis. Evidence, in other words, always underdetermines theory choice. Given a set of data points, we can draw infinitely many regressions that run through the dots. Each of them qualifies as a distinct hypothesis. In order to bridge the gap between evidence and theories, we often rely on "extra-evidential" considerations. We teach our students in laboratory courses to infer the appropriate lines by taking into account criteria like simplicity,

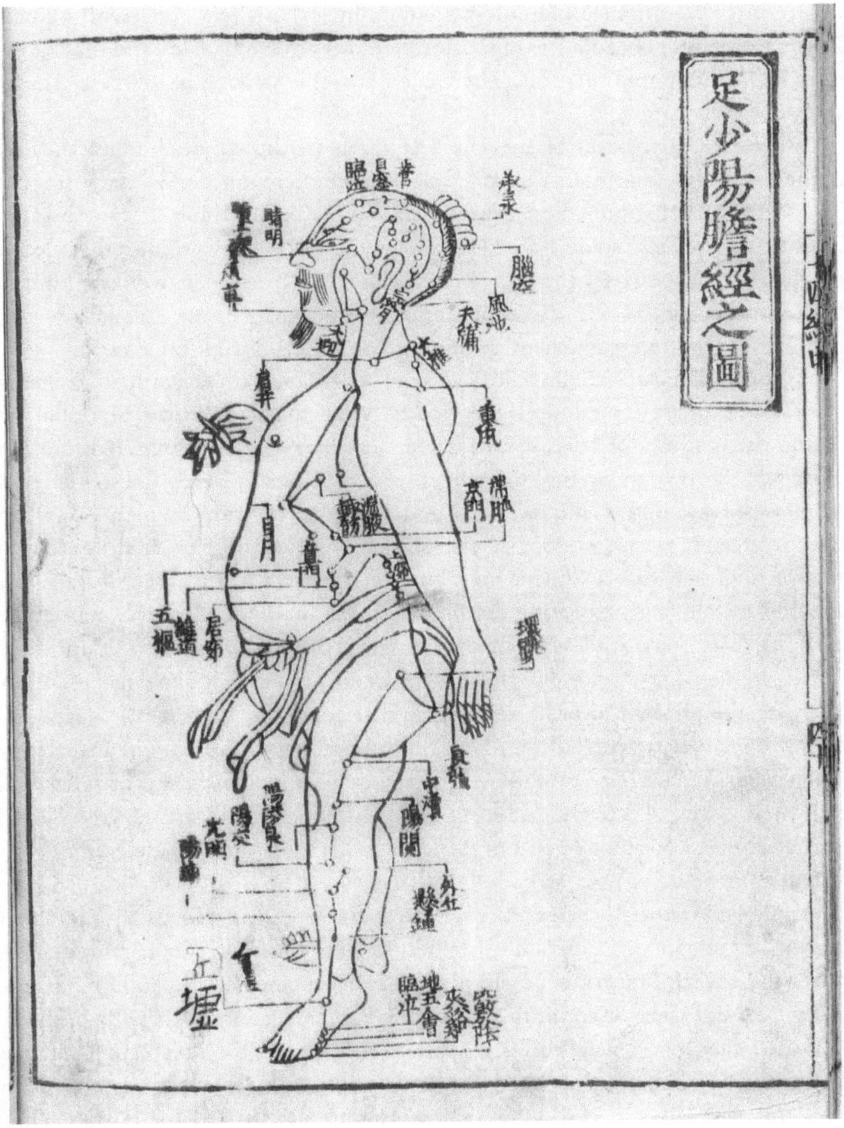

FIGURE 7.4 Hua Shou, Shisijing Fahui, 1341

Researchers have tried repeatedly to map Chinese medicine's meridian paths onto the Western understanding of human physiology. No account has been entirely satisfactory. See Longhurst (2010) for a critical discussion of past attempts and a new proposal. *Source:* Image from the National Library of Medicine.

computational convenience, and accuracy. These considerations are not supplied by the evidence; they are instead dictated by the values and pragmatic concerns of scientists. We might prefer a less accurate hypothesis (e.g., one with a lower R-squared value) because the regression requires fewer variables, and that allows us to make faster computations. The value of useable science, in this case, trumps the value of accuracy.

When we analyze data, often some data points are thrown out because they are outliers—likely experimental errors that we can safely ignore. We draw smooth lines between data points because there are no reasons to think that unobserved intermediate values would behave unexpectedly. And we avoid lines that clearly conflict with hypotheses that we already accepted. (In essence, we do a kind of Quinean revision to our scientific web of beliefs and choose conclusions and hypotheses that lead to the least amount of theoretical disruption.)

A good scientist somehow knows how to balance these competing values to draw the proper conclusion. Her ability is not magic, however. She operates within the confines of science, where years of training have hammered into her mind what sorts of theoretical inferences are acceptable. Learning the subtle art of theoretical reasoning is akin to learning social manners. And, like manners, when one violates the norms of good science, there is a price to be paid. A dissertation advisor might chastise a student for taking on a project that is just too wacky or too implausible (e.g., exploring the physiological effects of Mercury's retrograde motion). A graduate student in medicine whose dissertation flouts the norms of her discipline by, say, writing in the style of an epic poem will likely not get a job. Likewise, the pressure to produce research that generates "deliverables" leads scientists to set specific cut-off points for clinical trials, even though one can clearly achieve greater certainty by following patients for a longer period of time. As a community, we collectively decide that a trial lasting a sufficient length is good enough from an epistemic point of view. These decisions are the results of balancing different values: truth, safety, and urgency.

At the end of the day, scientists have to eat and pay their bills. As a professional pursuit, science cannot function if it raises the bar of justification so high that no reasonable amount of evidence can justify the acceptance of a hypothesis. Scientists would have starved to death a long time ago! We can insist that a hypothesis' ability to capture *all* data points be the only criterion for acceptance, but we would also forgo the practical benefits of elegant, simple, or useful hypotheses. To close the gap between data and hypotheses, we use values. And, logic and science cannot tell us which value to pick; only we can.

7.3 Contextual Values in Medicine: Values Outside of Scientific Reasoning

The claim that there are constitutive values that affect scientific reasoning is not particularly contentious. Pierre Duhem tells us that when a scientist confronts

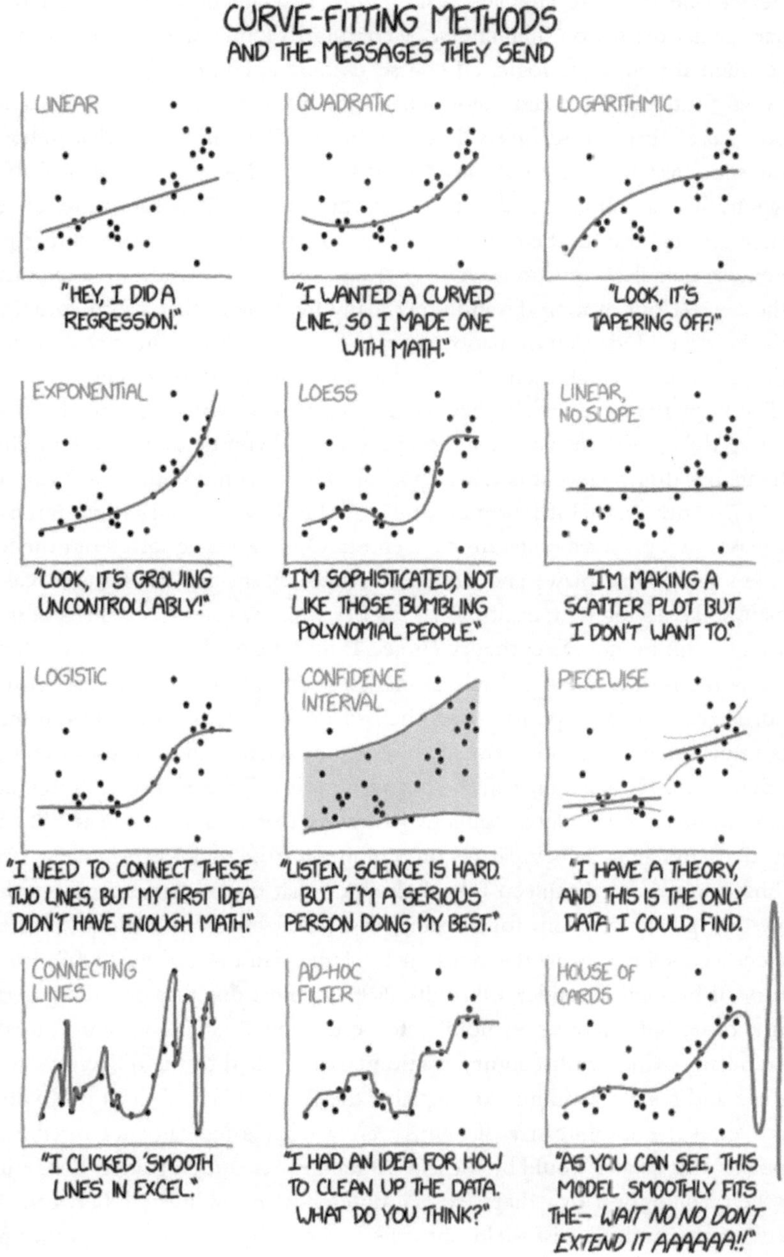

FIGURE 7.5 Curve Fitting

Source: From XKCD.com.

a false prediction, she has a choice to make: reject the hypothesis in question or reject one or more auxiliary assumptions that are needed to generate the experimental prediction. The choice, according to Duhem, is not guided by the experimental results and logic. Of course, Duhem attempts to pave over the gap between finite evidence and theory choice by introducing a notion of scientific "good sense" that tells scientists how to proceed. The difficulty is that unless we know more about what constitutes "good sense" and why it is a rational means of scientific reasoning, "good sense" is nothing more than the magic sauce of science. Analogously, in the case of confirmation, we see exactly the same gap. All the experimental observations we have do not uniquely identify one hypothesis as the correct one among the infinitely many hypotheses that are all compatible with the data. Underdetermination, in this sense, cuts both directions: evidence underdetermines which theory to reject and which theory to accept.

The hope for the positivists has always been that we will eventually be able to clean up the algorithms we use to accept or reject hypotheses. The task might be difficult, but they believe it is at least possible. However messy the inner workings of confirmation and falsification may turn out be, they are insulated from the values, biases, and practical concerns of scientists. Once we have sorted out the logic of science, personal biases and preferences like sexism and racism and real-life demands like paying rent, institutional politics, funding sources, conflicts of interests, and so on cannot affect theory choice. Either the evidence logically warrants the hypothesis or it doesn't. However racist a scientist might be, she cannot make veridical observation support a hypothesis if no support is rationally warranted. The impenetrable firewall between the logic of science and the social contexts of science ensures that values in the outside world will never bleed into scientific reasoning (even if the latter contains its own set of values). There is still some objectivity in science, albeit partly compromised by the underdeterminacy thesis.[5]

Philosophers like Kathleen Okruhlik argue that the underdeterminacy thesis allows for plenty of room for personal and social biases to infiltrate into theory choice.[6] Drawing on the research by Anne Fausto-Sterling (2008) on the history of biological gender, Okruhlik (1994) points out that prevailing gender norms often led scientists to hold onto certain hypotheses that conformed to these norms. Nineteenth-century craniometrists looked to the difference in size of male and female craniums to "explain" the intellectual inferiority of women. However, if the absolute size of brains were a reliable indicator for intelligence, elephants and whales would be the most intelligent creatures. Rather than rejecting their assumption that there exists a difference in intelligence between men and women, craniometrists held onto the hypothesis and looked for other possible explanations. Instead of absolute size, some theorized that it was the relative ratio of brain mass to body mass that mattered. But this explanation would entail the "unacceptable" conclusion that women were more intelligent than men and it was quickly rejected. Craniometrists then looked to the ratio of facial bones to cranial bones as the biological explanation for the inferior intelligence of women. This ratio, however, would put birds as the most intelligent animals.

German anatomist Emil Huschke (1854) argued in his *Schaedel, Hirn und Seele des Menschen und der Thiere nach Alter, Geschlecht und Race* (*Skull, Brain, and Soul of Man and of Animals by Age, Sex, and Race*) that the superiority of men's intellect was the result of a larger frontal lobe. Women, on the other hand, have larger parietal lobes (near the back of the head). This brain difference led him to propose that men should be referred to scientifically as "Homo frontalis" and women as "Homo parietalis." As new evidence emerged that the parietal lobe likely plays a greater role in one's intellect, researchers now claimed instead that women actually have smaller parietal lobes! It appears that regardless of what the evidence and the prediction show, the idea that men are more intelligent than women hangs around refusing to die.

As Quine and Duhum have noted, when confronted by observations that conflict with our experimental expectations, one always has a choice in terms of whether one rejects the cherished hypothesis or any of the auxiliaries that we assumed when we test a hypothesis. This choice, Okruhlik argues, can be dictated by our social mores, personal biases, and so on. Indeed, the entire scientific community can be blind to these assumptions, only to recognize their mistakes generations later.[7]

Okruhlik goes beyond pointing out how contextual values can affect theory choice. She argues that the very model of inference to the best explanation, even

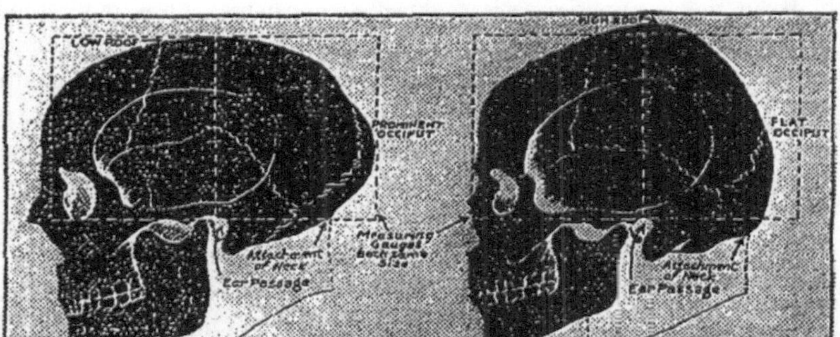

A comparison of the round-headed savage Prussian type of skull (on the right) and the gentle long-headed Teuton type (on the left), which Prof. Osborn says represents now only 10 per cent of Germans.

FIGURE 7.6 Craniology

Lest that one thinks craniology faded by the end of the 19th century, here is a 1918 Washington Post article titled "Science Explains the Prussian Ferocity of War." The rounded-headed "savage" Prussians inherited their barbarism from prehistorical racial mixing with "oriental hordes."

when the internal inferential logic is perfectly unaffected by social biases, will not be able to shed contextual values of the community at large. Recall that as an inferential rule, IBE tells us to accept the hypothesis that best explains the evidence. For instance, we believe that malaria is spread primarily by female mosquito bites. The hypothesis best explains our observations: we find the Plasmodium parasites in the salivary glands of female mosquitos, the use of mosquito nets in malaria-infested areas has significantly decreased incidents of malaria, etc. It would be fallacious, however, if IBE does not require there to be at last two hypotheses when we infer a hypothesis on the basis of evidence. Recall our gremlin example from Chapter 4: we do not want to accept the only hypothesis as the best in virtue of the fact that it is the sole hypothesis.

In order to avoid this absurdity, proponents of IBE have suggested that when inferring from observations to hypothesis, we must always consider at least two hypotheses. In this sense, IBE is always comparative: it involves comparisons and it only tells us, of the hypotheses in question, which one is more plausible. Okruhlik notes that so long as science engages in comparative judgments, rigorous and repeated applications of IBE cannot always shake out the biases that already existed in the hypotheses. She writes:

> [E]ven if we grant for the sake of argument that scientific method is itself free of contamination by non-cognitive factors and that the decision procedure operates perfectly [when we choose one theory over another], nothing in this procedure will insulate the content of science from sociological influences once we grant that these influences do affect theory generation. If our choice among rivals is irreducibly comparative, as it is on this model, then scientific methodology cannot guarantee (even on the most optimistic scenario) that the preferred theory is true—only that it is epistemically superior to the other actually available contenders. But if all these contenders have been affected by sociological factors, nothing in the appraisal machinery will completely "purify" the successful theory.
>
> *(1994, p. 34)*

We may have two hypotheses, with both assuming that women are less intelligent than men. An application of IBE would not "blow the whistle" on our hypotheses and tell us to reject both of them. Instead, it would tell us we should accept the hypothesis, however tainted by sexist presuppositions, that has greater explanatory power. This is putting aside that the application of IBE is itself affected by constitutive values.

The argument Okruhlik offers echoes some of the criticism of meritocracy. One might be tempted to argue that it is only fair to base college admissions on standardized tests to gauge the relative merits of applicants. Assume for the moment that standardized tests contain no biases. The problem with this approach is that if there exists widespread discrimination against a demographic (e.g., members of this group tend to go to schools that are poorly funded and the economic disparities are products of injustice), then a perfectly "fair" test would simply preserve the discrimination. Applicants who unjustly received an inferior education will do worse on the test. A pure meritocratic test cannot shake out preexisting injustices. In other words: garbage in, garbage out.

What Longino and Okruhlik show is that values can infect the workings of science at many points. Longino remains optimistic that although we cannot have the sort of objectivity that the positivists wanted, we can nevertheless have a kind of interactive objectivity (1990). Her idea is that if the participants of science (and the community at large) practice science in a transparent and democratic fashion with shared standards, we can call the results epistemically objective. She outlines four criteria that are necessary for science to be objective as a social practice:

(1) Forums for criticism: there must exist means by which scientific claims can be criticized;
(2) Public standards: there must be a set of shared values in evaluating scientific claims;
(3) Uptake of criticism: scientific claims must be sensitive to criticism; and
(4) Equality of intellectual authority: intellectual authority should be spread as widely as possible.

Echoing Mill's view on tolerance, Longino argues that as we include larger and more diverse viewpoints into scientific discourse, values and biases that each participant brings would be less dominant. Science will still be tainted with values, but they would not be of any one person's or even one community's values. They would be *our* values as a community at large.

In her later work, Longino extends her social epistemology of science to suggest that the ineliminable presence of values in science means that we have the opportunity to decide what kind of values we would like to guide our scientific practices. The interactive objectivity that she proposed earlier is but a recognition of our commitment to respecting stakeholders' say in the direction of science and how it affects all of us. It is ultimately our commitment to a kind of democratic ideal that supports her four criteria. Of course, democratic values are not the only values available. She argues that other values we hold dear ought to be embraced in scientific practice. In her essay, "Can There be a Feminist Science?" (1987), she argues that feminist values such as the critical unearthing of sexist presuppositions in our research can and should be a part of the values of science. Rather than running away from values, we ought to identify when values are implicitly or explicitly assumed in science. We do not need to stand idly by like mere spectators as value-laden science runs its course. We can take the reins and ensure that our science reflects our shared scientific, moral, and political values.[8]

7.4 Taking Charge of Medicine

The arguments explored in this chapter and the previous one suggest a pivot away from our ideal of a value-free medicine, both in clinical practices and in research. Following Longino's advice, we ought to be transparent about the sort of values we assume in medicine. And, most importantly, we can decide proactively what values we want to drive our practices. In some respects, this observation should strike us as ordinary and reasonable. Just about every social practice from education to political participation to allocation of social goods is infused and guided by values. The insistence that medicine be value-free is likely a relic held over from the positivist days, when the hope for the discovery of the "logic of science" and the reliance of the great firewall ruled the scientific and philosophical day. Philosophy in the past 50 years has raised some serious doubts that epistemology in general and science in particular can be value-free. The pertinent and urgent question for us is not how we can eliminate values from medicine, but what kind of values we would like to have in medicine.

Deciding which method we use to determine and to integrate values into medicine will not be a simple task. There are of course models that already exist. In the case of the allocation of social goods such as primary education, we decide as a community via democratic process how these resources should be distributed. The result might not be one that you like, but it will be (or at least should be) transparent and fair.[9] For now, at the very least, we need to acknowledge the ineliminable presence of values in medicine. Failing to do is not only a bad case of denial, it does a moral disservice to everyone involved.

Returning to the initial question we posed in the first chapter: what is the goal of medicine? Is it a science that seeks truth? Is it an art that makes us feel better? We can see answers emerging from our discussion of values—we want medicine to be guided by our values. Thus, the real question is what kind of values do we want? If values, as we have indicated, are not factive, then we need to decide collectively which of them we wish to live by. Our values can maximize social justice, quality of life, individual autonomy, social stability, and so on. As long as we can have open and informed discussions about values in other areas of our lives, we can surely do the same in medicine.

7.5 Science, Art, and a New Medicine

We began this book with a chapter discussing the scientific nature of medicine. The old Popperian falsifiability criterion that demarcates science from pseudo-science turns out to be implausible. To identify a pseudo-science according to Popper's criterion requires that the testing of hypotheses occur in isolation. Research by philosophers and historians of science have demonstrated that falsifiability is neither an accurate description of the actual practice of science, nor is it theoretically possible. Scientific holism, where theory choice is dictated by restoration of coherence in one's web of beliefs along the paths of least cognitive resistance, appears to be a far more plausible account of scientific practice. Quine thus writes:

> For my part I do, qua lay physicist, believe in physical objects and not in Homer's gods; and I consider it a scientific error to believe otherwise. But in point of epistemological footing, the physical objects and the gods differ only in degree and not in kind. Both sorts of entities enter our conceptions only as cultural posits. The myth of physical objects is epistemologically superior to most in that it has proved more efficacious than other myths as a device for working a manageable structure into the flux of experience.
>
> *(1951, p. 44)*

The "myth of physical object" is exactly as the name suggests: a tale that is woven out of our web of beliefs where revisions, additions, and eliminations of beliefs are dictated by criteria like simplicity and coherence with our other background beliefs (some of which supplied by cultural norms, per Okruhlik). There is nothing inherently special about empirical science; it is merely one of many possible ways we can make sense of the world around us and, for Quine, its preference is in its superior ability to organize our experiences.[10]

Quine was not the first philosopher to appreciate the specialness of science in terms of the instrumental values it offers. Science helps us makes sense of the world, delivers remarkable improvements to our quality of life, and gives us tools to bend nature to our will. American Pragmatists such as Charles Sanders Peirce and William James have advocated similar defenses. Seen from the pragmatist's point of view, science is special because it is useful. To be sure, it doesn't follow from this view that science offers nothing intrinsically valuable (valuable in and of itself). It has often been said that knowledge and truth are valuable for their own sake (like art for art's sake). Perhaps this is true.[11] But even if it were the case, it doesn't follow that the value of truths always trumps other intrinsic values. Typically, philosophers consider things like happiness, altruism, and autonomy to be intrinsically valuable. Things have instrumental values insofar as they deliver these intrinsic values. Suppose we add truths and knowledge to the list of intrinsically valuable things. When there is a conflict between whether to pursue happiness or truth, for instance, we still need to ask ourselves which one should win out. Given the holist's claims that science does not differ in kind from other ways of making sense of the world around us, medicine (as a science) becomes another pursuit that delivers valuable things. In the end, *we* get to decide what we care about and which tool to deploy to help us secure what we want.

All this might seem overly philosophical, but there are practical implications about how we conduct medicine. Once the bright line between science and non-science disappears, it becomes far harder to reject, say, certain therapies on the ground that they are unscientific. Whether prayers should be included in medical care is a question that cannot be answered *a priori* by merely looking at our definition of medicine. Rather, we need to ask ourselves whether the inclusion of prayers in medicine is congruent with things that we find valuable. Perhaps we include them because they bring about real improvement in patients' quality of life and we care more about that than our inability to square them with our commitment to empiricism. Alternatively, we might reject them because the clinical benefit does not outweigh the disruption to the tenets of empiricism and the myth of a physicalistic-based understanding of health and diseases. Regardless of how the debate concludes, one thing is clear: we should not ignore the agency we have in the matter. Philosophers' rejection of the specialness of science a la positivism with its robust objectivity and rationality does not lead us down the path of anything is as good as anything else. To draw that conclusion is to commit the fallacy of false dichotomy. Some ways of seeing and organizing our world are better than others in terms of their abilities to help us achieve our goals and in terms of their compatibility with our deep moral, political, and social values. A philosophically informed medicine is one that is tolerant, open-minded, transparent, and humble. These traits stem not from some vague commitment to political virtues; instead, they come from understanding the limits of what we can know.

The American philosopher Hilary Putnam, a neo-Pragmatist, concludes his short observation on the collapse of the fact-value distinction (1982) with this remark:

> So far, what I have said could be summarized by saying that if "values" seem a bit suspect from a narrowly scientific point of view, they have, at the very least, a lot of "companions of guilt": justification, coherence, simplicity, reference, truth, and so on, all exhibit the same problems that goodness and kindness do, from an epistemological point of view. None of them is reducible to physical notions: none of them is governed by syntactically precise rules. Rather than give them up all of them (which would be to abandon the ideas of thinking and talking), and rather than do what we are doing, which is to reject some—the ones which do not fit in with a narrow instrumentalist conception of rationality which itself lacks all intellectual justification—we should recognize that all values, including the cognitive ones, derive their authority from our idea of human flourishing and our idea of reason. These two ideas are interconnected: our image of an ideal theoretical intelligence is simply a part of our ideal of total human flourishing, as Plato and Aristotle saw.
>
> *(141)*

Medicine, like all human pursuits, ought to be grounded ultimately in how it affects us and what we value and care about. A pursuit that fetishizes one value over others misses the point of the endeavor entirely. Answering questions like

"Does medicine actually make us better off?", "What do we mean by 'better off' anyway?", and "What do we care about?" not only closes the perceived gap between medical sciences and the humanities, it also empowers us to take charge of our social institutions. Nothing is immutable. We just have to decide what we want.

Notes

1 For a theoretical and historic look at human experimentation on vulnerable populations, see Glenn (2015).

2 The distinction between constitutive values and contextual values mirrors the one between contexts of justification and contexts of discovery that the positivists endorsed. A central claim of classic positivism is that the social contexts that surround scientific practices—contexts of discovery—do not affect theoretical reasoning (e.g., if and how evidence supports a hypothesis). They call the latter the "context of justification."

3 Another fascinating place where values can enter into our scientific method is the adoption of conventions for rounding numbers. While most people tend to round up (e.g., 1.65 becomes 1.7), there are alternative systems. The banker system rounds to the closest *even* number (e.g., 1.5 would be rounded to 2 and 2.5 rounded to 2 as well). Which system one adopts often depends greatly on pragmatic factors. One might adopt a rounding down policy for taxation purposes so that tax payers always pay less taxes.

4 Again, we venture dangerously close to conflating metaphysics with epistemology. One might object that although we describe observations through the lenses of our theories, it doesn't follow that there is no fact of the matter about whether the stenosis is really there. The untrained viewer just doesn't notice it, but it is there all along in the venography. For applied domains like medicine, the question of whether seeing-as is a metaphysical or epistemic thesis is not that important. In both cases, one describes the observations in accordance with one's prior theories. The metaphysical or ontological status of the observation (e.g., is the stenosis *really* there?) matters little to the reality of practicing medicine.

5 It might be possible for the scientific community to agree to a set of non-logical conventions such as "Pick the simpler hypothesis if two hypotheses are both equally able to account for the data" (where we have some accepted definition of simplicity). Playing by the rules would thus ensure that individual biases are checked at the laboratory door by professional consensus. So, the argument goes.

6 Okruhlik uses the traditional terms "context of justification" and "context of discovery" instead of Longino's "constitutive values" and "contextual values." Although they are not perfectly overlapping, the two pairs are relatively similar.

7 One informative example is the removal of homosexuality as a mental illness from the second edition of the Diagnostic and Statistical Manual in 1972. See Drescher (2015) for a fascinating discussion of the history of the decision.

8 For those familiar with the unhealthy historic mix of politics and science (e.g., Lysenkoism), Longino's conclusion might set off alarm bells. These worries are not unreasonable. But, if what we have outlined so far is roughly correct, mixing values with science is unavoidable.

9 I can imagine a kind of Rawlsian argument to justify a democratic decision process where each stakeholder stands behind the veil of ignorance and determines what he or she wants.

10 If all coherent webs are nothing but competing myths, why should one not choose to believe in Homeric gods as opposed to quarks and muons? Epistemic voluntarism (i.e., being able to choose from a collection of worldviews as if one is shopping for pasta sauce in a supermarket) is a contentious thesis. One of the most obvious problems is

that when one chooses from a host of worldviews, one must do so from some point of view (or one must presuppose *a* worldview). There is no "view from nowhere," so to speak.

11 In a short paper, American philosopher Chase Wrenn (2017) uses a series of clever thought experiments to argue that truth is not intrinsically valuable and, even if it were, its value would be fairly low.

References

Drescher, J. (2015). Out of DSM: Depathologizing homosexuality. *Behavioral Sciences*, *5*(4), 565–575. doi:10.3390/bs5040565

Fausto-Sterling, A. (2008). *Myths of gender: Biological theories about women and men, revised edition*. New York, NY: Basic Books.

Glenn, J. E. (2015). Dehumanization, the symbolic gaze, and the production of biomedical knowledge. *Black knowledges/black struggles* (pp. 112–144). Liverpool: Liverpool University Press.

Huschke, E. (1854). *Schaedel, Hirn und Seele des Menschen und der Thiere nach Alter, Geschlecht und Race, dargestellt nach neuen Methoden und Untersuchungen*. Jena: Mauke.

Longhurst, J. C. (2010). Defining meridians: A modern basis of understanding. *Journal of Acupuncture and Meridian Studies*, *3*(2), 67–74. doi:https://doi.org/10.1016/S2005-2901(10)60014-3

Longino, H. E. (1983). Beyond "Bad Science": Skeptical reflections on the value-freedom of scientific inquiry. *Science, Technology, & Human Values*, *8*(1), 7–17. doi:10.1177/016224398300800103

Longino, H. E. (1987). Can there be a feminist science? *Hypatia*, *2*(3), 51–64.

Longino, H. E. (1990). *Science as social knowledge: Values and objectivity in scientific inquiry*. Princeton, NJ: Princeton University Press.

Magnusson, P., & Kastberg, R. (2017). Balloon venoplasty opens the road for an implantable defibrillator patient with complex stenosis. *Clinical Case Reports*, *5*(7), 1067–1071. doi:10.1002/ccr3.1002

Okruhlik, K. (1994). Gender and the biological sciences. *Canadian Journal of Philosophy*, *24*(sup1), 21–42.

Putnam, H. (1982). *Realism with a human face*. Cambridge, MA: Harvard University Press.

Quine, W.V. O. (1951). Two dogmas of empiricism. *Philosophical Review*, *60*(1), 20–43.

Wittgenstein, L. (1953). *Philosophical investigations* (Vol. 17). Oxford, UK: Wiley-Blackwell.

Wrenn, C. B. (2017). Truth is not (Very) intrinsically valuable. *Pacific Philosophical Quarterly*, *98*(1), 108–128.

Baker, M. (2016). 1,500 scientists lift the lid on reproducibility. *Nature*, *533*(7604), 452–454.

Ballou, S., Kaptchuk, T. J., Hirsch, W., Nee, J., Iturrino, J., Hall, K. T., . . . Davis, R. B. (2017). Open-label versus double-blind placebo treatment in irritable bowel syndrome: Study protocol for a randomized controlled trial. *Trials*, *18*(1), 234. doi:10.1186/s13063-017-1964-x

Begley, C. G., & Ellis, L. M. (2012). Raise standards for preclinical cancer research. *Nature*, *483*, 531. doi:10.1038/483531a

Bogaert, A. F., Skorska, M. N., Wang, C., Gabrie, J., MacNeil, A. J., Hoffarth, M. R., . . . Blanchard, R. (2017). Male homosexuality and maternal immune responsivity to the y-linked protein NLGN4Y. *Proceedings of the National Academy of Sciences*. doi:10.1073/pnas.1705895114

Burge, T. (1979). Individualism and the mental. *Midwest Studies in Philosophy, 4*(1), 73–122.

Drescher, J. (2015). Out of DSM: Depathologizing homosexuality. *Behavioral Sciences, 5*(4), 565–575. doi:10.3390/bs5040565

Feynman, R.P. (1990). *Q E D*: Penguin: *The strange theory of light and matter*. Princeton, NJ: Princeton University Press..

George, S. L., & Buyse, M. (2015). Data fraud in clinical trials. *Clinical investigation, 5*(2), 161–173. doi:10.4155/cli.14.116

Glenn, Jason E. (2015). Dehumanization, the symbolic gaze, and the production of biomedical knowledge. *Black Knowledges/Black Struggles* (pp. 112–144): Liverpool University Press.

Goodman, N. (1983). *Fact, fiction, and forecast* (4th ed.). Cambridge, MA: Harvard University Press.

Grant, D. C., & Harari, E. (2005). Psychoanalysis, science and the seductive theory of Karl Popper. *Australian and New Zealand Journal of Psychiatry, 39*(6), 446–452. doi:10.1080/j.1440-1614.2005.01602.x

Hájek, A. (2007). The reference class problem is your problem too. *Synthese, 156*(3), 563–585.

Hampl, J. S., & Hampl, W. S. (1997). Pellagra and the origin of a myth: Evidence from European literature and folklore. *Journal of the Royal Society of Medicine, 90*(11), 636–639.

Hawthorne, James. (1994). On the nature of bayesian convergence. PSA: *Proceedings of the Biennial Meeting of the Philosophy of Science Association*, 1994, 241–249.

Hume, David. (2000). *A treatise of human nature*: Oxford, UK: Oxford University Press.

Hume, David. (1998). *An inquiry concerning human understanding*. Oxford, UK: Oxford University Press.

James, William. (2014). The will to believe. In W. James (Ed.), *The will to believe: And other essays in popular philosophy* (pp. 1–31). Cambridge: Cambridge University Press.

Lexchin, J., Bero, L. A., Djulbegovic, B., & Clark, O. (2003). Pharmaceutical industry sponsorship and research outcome and quality: Systematic review. *BMJ: British Medical Journal, 326*(7400), 1167–1167.

Lipton, Peter. (2001). What good is an explanation? In G. Hon & S. Rakover (Eds.), *Explanation* (pp. 43–59): Springer Verlag.

Nuland, S. B. (2003). *The doctors' plague: Germs, childhood fever, and strange story of Ignaz Semmelweis*. New York: W.W. Norton.

Nuzzo, R. (2014). *Scientific method: Statistical errors. Nature*, 506, 150–152. doi:10.1038/506150a

Quill, T. E. (1991). Death and dignity. *New England Journal of Medicine, 324*(10), 691–694. doi:10.1056/nejm199103073241010

Quine, W.V. O. (1951). Two dogmas of empiricism. *Philosophical Review, 60*(1), 20–43.

Reznek, L. (1995). Dis-ease about kinds: Reply to D'Amico. *Journal of Medicine and Philosophy, 20*(5), 571–584. doi:10.1093/jmp/20.5.571

Ridge, M. (2014). *Impassioned belief*. Oxford, Oxford University Press.

Sakoulas, G., Wormser, G. P., Visintainer, P., Aronow, W. S., & Nadelman, R. B. (2009). Relationship between population density of attorneys and prevalence of methicillin-resistant staphylococcus aureus: Is medical-legal pressure on physicians a driving force behind the development of antibiotic resistance? *American Journal of Therapeutics, 16*(5).

Silva, J. C., Loreto, E. L., & Clark, J. B. (2004). Factors that affect the horizontal transfer of transposable elements. *Current Issues in Molecular Biology, 6*(1), 57–71.

The Open Science Collaboration. (2015). Estimating the reproducibility of psychological science. *Science, 349*(6251).

Tulodziecki, D. (2013). Shattering the myth of Semmelweis. *Philosophy of Science, 80*(5), 1065–1075.

Williams, G. C. (1957). Pleiotropy, natural selection, and the evolution of senescence. *Evolution, 11*(4), 398–411. doi:10.2307/2406060

Wrenn, C. B. (2017). Truth is not (Very) intrinsically valuable. *Pacific Philosophical Quarterly, 98*(1), 108–128.

INDEX